Keto Diet for Beginners

The Newest Guide to Understand the Basic Principles about Ketogenic Diet. Find Out How You Can Get Into Ketosis to Lose Weight Fast

Table of Contents

Chapter 1: Introduction to Keto Diet

At the beginning of every year, and every day in between, people hear about a new diet, detox plan, or gym membership that promises to be the secret to a successful year or a healthy life. Sometimes, it seems like the whole world is trying to get rid of a few extra pounds as fast as possible. Often people are willing to try anything that sounds remotely promising.

Enter the keto diet. This diet plan is one of the hottest trends currently. Interestingly, its origins date back to the 1920s as a treatment plan for childhood epilepsy. Due to its overwhelming popularity and success rate, many people still use it to deal with this condition today.

According to some studies, people who follow this diet experience up to 40% fewer epileptic seizures. Its use, however, is more common in the generally healthy population seeking to get more out of life or drop a few pounds. This diet plan promises a wide range of benefits from increased mental focus to faster weight loss.

The keto diet aims to decrease insulin and blood sugar levels by shifting the body's metabolism to burn fat more effectively to generate energy, which leads to the production of ketones. In addition, proponents of this diet plan insist that it can help people lose weight quite fast, which is one of the reasons why it is so popular.

However, to determine whether this diet plan is good for them, people need to learn as much as possible about the keto diet. They need to determine whether science backs it before joining the cause and adopting it into their lifestyle.

1.1 What Is the Keto Diet Plan?

The word keto comes from the fact that this diet plan drives the body to produce ketones, which are tiny energy/fuel molecules. The body turns to this fuel source when the level of blood sugar is low. The human brain is a constantly hungry organ that needs a lot of energy, which is understandable given the work it does every second. However, it cannot run on fat; rather, it needs glucose or ketones.

This diet plan consists of consuming food that is low in carbohydrates, moderate in protein, and significantly high in fat. Actually, according to some keto diet variations, the fat content should make up to 80% of a person's daily calories. The carbohydrates, on the other hand, should be less than 5% of the calories. Protein should contribute between 15% and 20% of the calories.

It is easy to see why many people are apprehensive about this diet plan. The keto diet drastically departs from the generally accepted macronutrient distribution of 10% to 35% fat, 45% to 65% carbs, and 20% to 35% protein. However, the most important aspect of this diet is the normal and natural process known as ketosis.

The healthy human body runs quite well on the glucose produced when the body burns or breaks down carbohydrates. Actually, the human body prefers to generate energy through the breakdown of carbohydrates. However, when a person is hungry or cutting back on carbohydrates, his/her body will seek other sources of energy.

Fat is an alternative source of energy for the body. When a person's blood sugar is low because he/she is not feeding his/her body with carbohydrates, his/her cells will release fat and flood the liver. Consequently, the liver will turn the fat into ketone bodies, which the body will use as its secondary energy source.

In other words, the ketogenic diet aims to substitute the body's primary sources of energy with fats. Actually, this process is surprisingly efficient, which is why it leads to weight loss and other health benefits. Another subtle benefit of this diet plan is that one will have a constant supply of energy and feel hungry less often.

Consequently, one will feel focused and sharp all day. As stated earlier, the keto diet helps decrease insulin and blood sugar levels. Sugar, however, is the brain's main fuel or food. Fortunately, ketones produced by the liver from fat will feed the brain. Most people who follow this diet plan insist it is quite safe.

Nevertheless, the ketogenic diet is still controversial. Actually, three groups of people should keep away from this diet. These are breastfeeding women, people with high blood pressure taking antihypertensive medication, and people with diabetes who take insulin. Before adopting this diet, people in these situations should seek their doctors' advice.

People on a keto diet force their bodies to run on fat, essentially, their bodies burn fat 24 hours a day, seven days a week, as long as they are following this diet plan religiously. The fastest way to get the body into a state of ketosis is through fasting. However, it is extremely difficult to fast for several days.

This is where the keto diet comes in handy. This diet plan helps the body reach this state surprisingly fast, and people can adopt and follow it indefinitely. A typical ketogenic diet consists of foods such as butter, meat, cheese, fish, eggs, heavy cream, avocado, oils, seeds, nuts, and low-carb green veggies.

Looking at this list, one will notice that it does not include people's favorite carbohydrate-rich foods such as fruits, grains, cereals, rice, milk, beans, sweets, potatoes, and even some veggies.

1.2 The Science of Keto

Every year, new diet fads rise and fall with little to commend them. Nothing new there; however, the keto diet has been around for a remarkably long time and continues to gain popularity because of the science behind it. Many prominent medical professionals believe in the benefits of ketosis, which is reason enough for one to take a closer look at this diet.

After years of trying any weight loss diets, most overweight individuals come to believe that nothing makes a difference. They only lose some weight if they consume fewer calories than they used to, but when they do this, then they feel hungry all the time, which causes them to binge eat on certain occasions. When such individuals learn about the ketogenic diet, few can resist its attraction.

The concept behind this diet plan makes a lot of sense. The weirdly named ketone bodies are tiny molecules that serve as the natural back-up fuel supply for the body when glucose is in short supply. As stated earlier, people normally enter ketosis when they starve themselves for several days at a time.

Ketosis is the state where ketone bodies build up in the bloodstream. When the body reaches ketosis, metabolism switches to fat-burning to convert accumulated fat molecules into ketone bodies, which help power the brain and muscles. Being in a state of ketosis, therefore, sounds like an awesome way to get rid of excess fat.

Not eating for days, on the other hand, is not something most people would be willing to do. Fortunately, the keto diet seems to be the answer to this dilemma. People do not need to starve themselves to reach ketosis. Instead, all they need to do is drastically reduce the carbohydrates in their diet, and this includes refined carbs, complex carbs, as well as starches.

When the body lacks a source of glucose, it has to go into a state of ketosis since the brain needs fuel in the form of either glucose or ketone bodies to function and survive. Therefore, no matter how much fat or protein one eats, the body will still need to break down fat to ketone bodies to produce the fuel it needs.

As earlier stated, there are many variations of the keto diet. All of them, however, aim to switch the body's metabolism to ketosis. Actually, the keto diets doing the rounds out there are not the only ones or the first to do that. The Atkins diet, for example, rose to prominence a few decades ago and helped many people lose weight.

The Atkins diet, in reality, is another variation of the keto diet since it removes carbohydrates from the diet and substitutes them with protein. Interestingly, followers of this diet discovered that they felt less hungry than they feared, which means that the calories from increased protein intake made the feel satisfied for longer.

When one is feeling full, one will eat less, which will translate to significant weight loss. The Atkins diet, however, has certain side effects for people who follow it for an extended period. The most troubling of these side effects is its impact on the balance of nitrogen from the consumption of too much protein.

For example, there is an increased risk of dehydration for those who adhere to the Atkins diet. In serious cases, the need to get rid of excess nitrogen as urine leads to the formation of kidney stones. In a certain sense, the keto diet is the 21st-century version of the Atkins diet. Instead of replacing carbohydrates with protein, the keto diet replaces them with fats.

The regimen of a typical Atkins diet consisted of less than 5% of calories from carbohydrates, 25% from fats, and about 75% from protein. The modern keto diet regimen, in contrast, suggests 25% of calories from protein, less than 5% from carbohydrates, and about 75% from fats.

Since the intake of protein in the keto diet is the same as the recommended protein intake in a typical balanced diet, it neatly sidesteps the side effects resulting from nitrogen imbalance. However, the recommended fat intake in the keto diet is a huge concern for many people.

It seems more than a bit ironic that it advocates for people who want to get rid of excess fat to include more fats in their diet. To many people, it seems quite unhealthy. To help understand this conundrum, consider the case if the lipid profiles of the brave individuals who explore and cross the Antarctic on foot while dragging sleds packed with food and supplies.

To achieve this feat, they need to take food with a very high calorie to weight ratio. Essentially, this means eating a lot of butter. It takes several months to cross the continent on foot, which means living on an all-butter diet for months. Interestingly, after months on this diet, the level of bad cholesterol in their bodies, known as LDL-cholesterol, actually decreases significantly.

This may surprise many people, but it is not as surprising as it sounds. When the body goes into ketosis, it moves fats towards the liver, where the transformation of fats into ketone bodies happens, which is the work of HDL-cholesterol. Usually, LDL-cholesterol transports excess fat from the liver to deposits in different parts of the body.

Essentially, this type of cholesterol moves fat in the opposite direction. In ketosis, therefore, no matter how much fat one is consuming, one will have a lipid profile usually considered healthier. In other words, one will have lower LDL and higher HDL, which is quite remarkable.

However, as discussed earlier, one of the benefits of following the Atkins diet was reduced feelings of hunger due to the sustaining power of protein. People often wonder how the keto diet can achieve this without increasing the protein content of their diet. As it turns out, reduced hunger stems from the state of ketosis itself.

In a certain sense, it might not matter how one achieves this state. Therefore, theoretically, science seems to back up the modern keto diet. However, it would be somewhat interesting to imagine how it would feel to follow the keto diet in place of the commonly touted, calorie-deficient, low-everything diet.

Consider a man weighing 195 pounds on a 5-foot, 9-inch frame at the beginning of the year. This would put his body mass index at about 30, which is quite close to being obese. Anyway, on the first day of the year, he reads about the keto diet, does some research, and decides to try it.

He purchases one of the deliciously sounding cookbooks from Amazon and begins the keto journey. His intake of carbohydrates immediately falls below 5%, which means, among other things, eating a rib-eye steak topped with chili-butter, followed with cheese and scrambled eggs in the morning. This sounds somewhat awesome.

Anyway, people who believe that fats are an important ingredient in great tasting food should find the keto diet quite appealing and easy to follow. This man usually works out for 30 minutes each day on a rowing machine. To improve the effectiveness of his new diet, he decides to increase his workout time to 45 minutes.

This workout will help get rid of excess carbohydrates in his body stored as glycogen in the liver, which will release quickly to power his muscles. Within 2 days, he reaches ketosis. Using urine dipsticks, he determines that his ketone body level indicates a state of deep ketosis.

The level of ketone bodies stayed constant for more than a month while he enjoyed the culinary delights of meals such as cream pork stroganoff accompanied by zucchini ribbons sour cream and avocado dressings, and burgers. Essentially, he was eating three fat-rich meals each day.

In this example, it is important to look at the benefits he enjoyed before looking at any disadvantages. Once he went into a state of ketosis a few days on, he founds that he was never hungry. Essentially, he stopped snacking between meals as he usually did. Actually, he found himself thinking less about eating.

Soon, missing lunch altogether by accident became something quite normal. There was a significant improvement in his focus and concentration as well, in addition to having more energy, which also increased his productivity. In other words, using his back-up batteries, which are the tiny ketone bodies, seemed to be better than using carbohydrates for fuel.

There is a good reason why this might happen, especially for a chubby individual like the person in this example. Essentially, the ketone levels never decline. By contrast, when people eat carbohydrate-rich foods, the metabolism system immediately turns the excess carbohydrates into fat. In a sense, it stores it for a rainy day.

Therefore, after eating a carbohydrate-rich meal, a person's blood glucose level starts to decrease a few hours after, which triggers feelings of hunger and the urge to eat again. In addition, it also triggers a sense of declining concentration and energy, which carb-eaters and late afternoon dippers know so well.

Going back to the hypothetical man in the example above, eating less actually led to a significant loss of weight. For this example, based on a testimonial from the real individual, he lost 10 pounds in less than a month, mostly from unhealthy-looking and unattractive fat deposits on his body.

According to his testimonial, his waistline decreased by two notches, which is twice as much as his previous diet achieved by keeping hi constantly hungry. In addition, the keto diet brought other unexpected benefits as well. The amount of plaque on his teeth, for example, reduced quite significantly, maybe because carbohydrates need to feed off dietary carbohydrates.

When it comes to the downside of the keto diet, at least according to him, there were just a few. The first is about staying away from carbohydrates, keeping them below 5% proved to be quite challenging after a couple of weeks. He had to check the content of carbohydrates in everything he ate, which was difficult because he found them in almost everything he chose to eat.

Eating out was also a challenge, not to mention having to attend dinner parties at a family member or friend's house unless they were unusually accommodating. As a result, planning and preparing food took on a new level of significance and demand for his resources and time than previously.

Secondly is the issue of accurate portion control. Since the keto diet includes high-fat meals with high-calorie content, he often feared he would unintentionally consume too many calories. To lose weight people need to eat fewer calories than they need. Even the ketogenic diet cannot break this law.

The last downside was a bit easier to avoid. While following the keto diet, it is difficult to get enough fiber mainly because most of the fiber sources commonly available also contain carbohydrates. Essentially, since fiber is an indigestible or insoluble carbohydrate polymer, it naturally contains digestible carbohydrates. His solution was to take a fiber supplement.

If this man were to conduct an experiment to determine the impact of eating some carbs after following a carbohydrate-free diet for a month, just a small portion of carbohydrates would immediately kill ketosis. He would then need to re-establish ketosis after one moment of weakness. Following the keto diet, therefore, requires Zen-like discipline.

This experiment shows that ketosis is difficult and slow to establish, but very easy to turn off. Scientists call this phenomenon hysteresis. There are good reasons for this. Although carbohydrates and glucose good sources of fuel, they can damage the proteins that make up the body's tissues and cells.

When the levels of glucose go up too much, this tissue and cell damage may be irreversible, which can happen in diabetes. To prevent this from happening, the body produces insulin as soon as the levels of blood glucose start to go up. Insulin limits glucose levels in the blood by instructing the liver to turn excess glucose into fat.

In the process, however, insulin kills ketosis, which is why ketosis ends so quickly when people following the keto diet slip up. Nowadays, there is unlimited availability of calories.

The body stores every oz. of excess carbohydrates as fat. Without establishing ketosis, the body will not re-assess these fat deposits when glucose runs out; instead, one will simply feel hungry. With fast-food joints around every corner, it is extremely tempting to refuel with carbohydrates again.

As stated earlier, one reason why people lose weight while on a keto diet is that feelings of hunger go way down, which forces more fat out of fat deposits for energy than the fat that goes in. Without spikes in insulin, the body takes advantage of leptin-induced satiety ore easily.

The keto diet also helps people wean off dopamine addiction caused by spiking blood sugar, which raises HDL and reduces LDL and triglycerides in obese people. However, people who want to try the keto diet should first discuss it with their doctor to determine whether it is good for them.

1.3 Ketogenic Diet and Diabetes

The Ketogenic diet is something that makes headlines these days, and that's because approvals by celebrities and supermodels have pushed it into popular culture. However, one of the questions being asked is,"Is the ketogenic diet plan effective for people with diabetes?"

Medically, the Ketogenic diet is not highly recommended for people with type 1 diabetes' however, in terms of the management of type 2 diabetes, there is no straightforward answer.

Some data shows that the ketogenic diet might be helpful, while others like a study on Nutrients published in September 2016, highlights the significance of whole grains as a dietary requirement for people living with diabetes - an unacceptable category of food in the keto diet.

Though the Ketogenic diet comes with a lot of potential benefits for the management of diabetes, a lot of discipline and commitment is required in other to reap the rewards. Thus, if you're someone suffering from diabetes, it is important to explore the following questions in other to ascertain whether it's right for you.

What exactly are the health benefits of a Keto Diet for Diabetes?

According to Lori Zanini, RD, CDE, the author of *Eat What You Love* Diabetes Cookbook, if you are trying to manage type 2 diabetes, this is how the ketogenic diet may help, "With a higher protein and fat intake, individuals may feel less hungry and are often able to lose weight, since protein and fat take longer to digest than carbohydrates." It also helps to boost and maintain energy levels.

The ketogenic diet also contains other possible benefits. For example, a September 2016 review posits that a Keto diet may improve A1C test results for people with diabetes (A result that shows average blood sugar levels within 3 months) better than low-calorie diets. The diet can also help reduce triglycerides better than a low-fat diet, which is beneficial for diabetes patients that are exposed to a higher risk for heart disease.

In addition, a keto diet is likely to be three times more efficient for weight loss than a low-fat diet - impressive because the loss of even five to ten percent of total body weight can come with health benefits such as improved blood pressure, cholesterol, and blood sugar mitigation (as stated by the Center for Disease Control and Prevention). Furthermore, the European Journal of Clinical

Nutrition in August 2013 published a review that posited that a Keto diet might be capable of controlling blood sugar levels and improving cholesterol levels.

Is the Keto diet the most effecting eating approach for Type 2 Diabetes?

Several modern research studies support the use of the ketogenic diet in the management of diabetes, and some hospitals have gone as far as implementing therapeutic keto programs. Virta Health, which offers a telemedicine lifestyle and diet program, has projected research that shows that embracing online support may help diabetic patients lower their A1C, lose weight and get off diabetes medication more successfully than the American Diabetes Association recommended the diet. Diabetes Therapy published the study in February 2018.

However, it is important to understand that the Keto diet isn't the best possible path for every diabetic patient. Some studies project other plans like the Mediterranean diet - which is rich in vegetables, lean meats, fruits, nuts, whole grains, olive oil, and fish- to be more suited for diabetic patients. In the April 2014 issue of the Nutrients, a published review posited that the Mediterranean diet helps to lower the risk of developing type 2 Diabetes.

In the January issue of Diabetes Care, a randomized controlled trial posited that adherence to a Mediterranean diet without any calorie ceiling might help prevent diabetes. The diet plan may also help people already inflicted with the sickness. The review also quoted some studies that linked the Mediterranean diet with better blood sugar control.

There are risks associated with the Keto diet. In 2016, the Journal of Obesity and Eating Disorders published a study that posits that type 2 diabetic patients who take oral medication to reduce their blood sugar may be prone to low blood sugar or hypoglycemia when following a keto diet. Also, a keto diet can lead to side effects like chills, fever, fast heartbeat, excessive hunger and thirst, confusion, fatigue, headache, nausea, dizziness, and bad breath, etc.

If you are suffering from Type 2 Diabetes, what is the best way to start a Keto Diet?

If you're living with type 2 diabetes, it is advisable to check in with your medical support team before you explore the Keto diet plan. Also, it is important to slowly implement the diet, gradually reducing carbs, because radical reductions may cause low blood sugar or hypoglycemia, especially for people on insulin or oral diabetes medications. Sylvia White, RD, CDE, a nurse In Memphis, Tennessee, says, "If your blood sugar level dips, glucagon, the emergency medication, might not even be able to boost it."

She went on to stress the need for regular checks on ketone and blood sugar levels to ward off serious side effects. "It is important to do so to avoid diabetic ketoacidosis. Some early symptoms of diabetic ketoacidosis include consistent high ketone levels, high blood sugar, frequent urination, dry mouth, vomiting, and nausea. These complications can result in a diabetic coma.

It is also important to consume a balance of nutrients, especially fiber, minerals, vitamins, and others - as well as the right amount of healthy keto-friendly fats and calories. Generally, healthy fats include omega-3s and monounsaturated fats, which are known to improve cholesterol levels and reduce inflammation. Consume sunflower seeds, peanut butter, almonds, and avocados for monounsaturated fats, and a fatty fish like salmon for omega-3s.

If you're confused, reach out to your dietician, because most times people only focus on what not to eat, without paying attention to foods that should be included in their diets, including lean proteins, healthy monounsaturated fats, vegetables, and many more.

How do you stick to the low carb count on the Keto Diet?

No matter how you look at it, it's not an easy task to eat just twenty to sixty grams of carbs per day (the permitted amount of carbs on the keto diet). Thus, for people to observe this rigid guideline, they need to change the food they eat and their entire lifestyle.

Typical foods that constitute the American diet like milkshakes, Big Macs, and for-long subs, don't fit into the ketogenic diet plan - also, foods known as staples of a balanced diet such as whole-grain bread and sweet potatoes may need to be controlled. These modifications can be hard to execute, even for people already eating healthy diets. A practice that comes in handy is tracking the food you eat. You can either use apps on your smartphone or with a paper food diary.

The plan doesn't allow you to take days off. You have to be disciplined if you intend to achieve results - or else you'll just be eating a high-protein, high-fat diet.

Is the Keto diet safe for everyone who has Type 2 Diabetes?

The ketogenic diet is not safe for everyone with Type 2 diabetes; it is particularly bad for people that have already developed kidney issues because then, protein intake has to be limited.

People with type 1 diabetes also need to be wary of the keto diet. The American Diabetes Association warns that Ketones (synthesized during ketosis) are mainly a risk factor for DKA, which is prominent in people with type 1 diabetic patients than type 2 diabetic patients.

It is also important to diligently look out for other possible symptoms of DKA.

Furthermore, another set of people that should be wary of the Keto diet are those with a history of heart disease. During the initial stages of the Keto diet, cholesterol levels tend to increase and this can increase the risk of heart disease. Also, yo-yo dieting, which can easily occur on a keto diet plan, is capable of straining the heart, possibly causing a heart attack or stroke.

It is important to work with a dietician or doctor to work out the right diet plan for you, especially if you have a history of struggling with an eating disorder. Irrespective of what you've heard or read on the internet, you have to understand that a history of binge eating disorder and the Keto diet do no match at all. The restrictions imposed by the ketogenic diet on carbs increases the risks of compulsive overeating, bingeing, and other eating disorders.

1.4 Advantages of the Keto Diet

In the beginning, the ketogenic diet can be quite overwhelming. Before people give it a go, they need to understand what it involves, how the diet works, and, most importantly, what doctors and nutritionists think about the ketogenic diet. According to many people who follow the keto diet plan, it provides impressive results within a very short time.

Research also suggests that the keto diet may even improve workout performance in athletes and help them lose body fat while maintaining muscle mass. However, it is important to note that conflicting evidence exists to support these claims. Some experts, for example, express concerns about the sustainability of this diet plan, as well as its long-term effects on the body.

Some of the common advantages of the keto diet include:

1. Quick weight loss
2. Tons of online recipes and resources
3. Ability to boost satiety
4. Improved athletic performance in certain people
5. Reduced abdominal fat
6. Ay improve health markers like cholesterol levels, triglyceride, and blood pressure

1.5 Mechanism of Keto Diet

The keto diet restricts the intake of proteins and especially carbohydrates while encouraging the consumption of fat. For several decades, doctors have been using this diet plan in the management and treatment of drug-resistant epilepsy. This is because its action mechanism leads to changes in ketone levels and other substances, thereby reducing the frequency of seizures.

- **Seizure Pathophysiology**

The brain has a complex network of neurons that transmit signals and nerve impulses. These transmitters play a critical role in the dissemination of these nerve impulses, which carry messages across the neuron synapse. Neurotransmitters are inhibitory or excitatory based on their effect on the triggering of impulses.

A common excitatory neurotransmitter is a glutamate, which aids the distribution of impulses. On the other hand, GABA serves to inhibit nerve impulses. Any imbalance between the brain's neurotransmitters causes a seizure, especially due to the firing of too many nervous messages and over-excitement of the nerves.

Therefore, GABA helps to control the frequency of epileptic seizures, while anticonvulsant medication helps to boost inhibitory neurotransmitters. Scientists do not know the keto diet's precise mechanism; however, they propose several possible explanations.

Many changes take place in the brain and body because of the keto diet. However, science is yet to identify the change that leads to the anticonvulsant effect. That said, the action mechanism of most pharmacological anticonvulsant medication is similarly mysterious.

The most important aspect of the keto diet is the drastic restriction of carbohydrates from the diet. To compensate for this reduction, the conversion of fatty acids into sources of fuel takes place through oxidation in the mitochondria. The lack of carbohydrates in the diet leads to the absence of glucose.

Acetone, acetoacetate, and hydroxybutyrate, which are ketone bodies, synthesize and pass through the blood-brain barrier to provide an alternative energy source for the brain. Scientists think they possess anticonvulsant properties needed to prevent seizures in test animals.

The propagation of nerve messages and stabilization of neurons may happen because of the ketone bodies' efficiency as a source of fuel. As the body adapts to the conversion of fat to produce ketone bodies for energy, the increase in the number of mitochondria takes place.

Both the keto diet and pharmacological anticonvulsants work because of their ability to suppress seizures. Unlike anticonvulsant medication, however, the keto diet seems to have anti-epileptogenic properties and the ability to hinder the progress of epilepsy, at least according to a study of rats.

There are several other theories about the keto diet's action mechanism, such as hypoglycemia, electrolyte changes, and systemic acidosis, which is increased blood acidity. However, science is yet to prove the accuracy of most of these theories. In addition, some evidence suggests that these hypotheses may not have anything to do with the diet's mechanism.

Within the past twenty years or so, interest in determining the therapeutic mechanism of the keto diet has been growing steadily. Fortunately, modern advances in the scientific and medical fields are yielding critical insight into the biochemical basis of many brain functions, both pathologic and normal.

Some of the metabolic changes likely connected to the keto diet's anticonvulsant properties include increased bioenergetics reserves, increased fatty acid levels, reduced glucose levels, and ketosis.

According to some experts in the field of neuroscience, some of the effects induced by the keto diet may include GABA neurotransmission and enhanced purinergic, sensitive potassium channel modulation, and boosted brain-derived neurotropic factor expression because of glycolytic limitation.

More importantly, in addition to its use as an anticonvulsant, the keto diet may also promote neuroprotective properties, which can help boost the clinical potential of the diet as an illness-prevention approach or intervention.

Since scientific evidence proves that changes in diet can trigger a wide range of complex metabolic alterations, future scientific research should reveal a more detailed framework for the keto diet mechanism in action, which will allow for the formulation of an improved offering with fewer side effects for a wide range of physical disorders.

Some scientists proposed the modulation of the levels of biogenetic monoamine as a plausible action mechanism for the anticonvulsant properties of the keto diet. The specific workings underlying such properties, however, remain unclear. Norepinephrine levels in test animals seem to show an increase in rats consuming this diet.

When researchers inhibited the transport of norepinephrine, there was no observable benefit from the keto diet. This seems to suggest the need for a noradrenergic system for the neuroprotective properties of the ketogenic diet to take place. From this brief discussion, it is clear to see the complexity of the keto diet's mechanism of action.

1.6 Common Mistakes of Keto

The hottest diet last year, which is the ketogenic diet, is only gaining momentum this year. It attracts more than one million searches on Google each month, which is a testament to its popularity. However, this popularity tends to make people who want to try it out make various mistakes.

Unfortunately, people tend to jump headlong into any weight loss and wellness diet that promises amazing results without doing adequate research to determine whether the diet is right for them. This is also true when it comes to the keto diet. It is difficult to know what to expect when one decides to follow the keto diet without proper research.

The most important thing to understand about this low-carb, high-fat diet is that it is extremely restrictive; therefore, getting it right can be quite difficult. For example, in addition to the obvious carbohydrates, people who want to adopt this diet need to avoid starchy vegetables and limit grains, fruits, sweets, and juices.

In addition, they will need to bulk up on fats, according to the recommended keto food list. By doing this, they will go into ketosis within a very short time, which, as discussed earlier, is the metabolic state that forces their bodies to burn fat to generate fuel, instead of burning carbohydrates. In most cases, this will speed up their weight-loss goals.

Since carbohydrates are in just about everything people eat today and fats come in several different forms, it is easy to make mistakes, especially if one does not know much about the ketogenic lifestyle. At this point, it is important to understand that not all fats are healthy.

To live the keto lifestyle safely, one needs to understand the common mistakes people make, including:

1. **Increasing Fat Intake and reducing Carbohydrate Intake too Quickly and too Much**

One day, one is eating cereal in the morning, sandwiches at lunch, and pasta for dinner. Suddenly, having decided to adopt the keto diet, one will need to consume less than 20 grams of carbohydrates every day, based on the starting amount recommended by the keto diet. This is harder to achieve than it sounds.

A medium apple, for example, contains approximately 25 grams of carbohydrates. This is a good point of reference for people who decide to follow the keto diet. Essentially, this diet requires drastic dietary and lifestyle changes. Therefore, it is important to ease into the diet. Before adopting this diet fully, people should begin by decreasing their carbohydrates intake gradually, instead of doing it cold turkey.

2. **Failing to Drink Adequate Water**

When most people start weight loss or wellness diets, including the keto diet, they tend to focus on what they are eating and forget about what they are drinking. People on the ketogenic diet have an increased risk of dehydration due to the extreme decrease in their carbohydrate intake.

This can easily lead to a shift in electrolyte and fluid balance. The body stores carbohydrates along with water; therefore, as the deposits of carbohydrates in the body run dry, excess water in the body also depletes. In addition, the body gets rid of excess ketones through urine, which depletes sodium and water from the body.

Therefore, it is important to drink a lot of water to prevent dehydration. When one wakes up, for example, one should drink a glass of water and sip water regularly throughout the day, which will help one reach the goal of drinking half of one's body weight in oz. of water every day.

3. **Failing to Prepare for the Keto Flu**

As one's body transitions from a carbohydrate engine to a fat engine, one might experience the keto flu, which comes with flu-like symptoms such as fatigue, body aches, nausea, and cramps. This often happens during the first couple of weeks; however, these symptoms do not affect everyone who adopts this diet.

People who lack knowledge about the keto diet and fail to prepare themselves for these symptoms often think there is something very wrong, which makes them give up on the diet altogether.

However, such people can overcome these symptoms by planning their prepping and meal preparation in advance. It is also wise to eat foods rich in sodium, magnesium, and potassium, in addition to drinking water to help deal with any negative symptoms of this diet.

Other common mistakes people make when they decide to adopt the keto diet include:

- Failing to eat foods rich in omega-3 fatty acids
- Failing to salt their food adequately
- Failing to consult their doctor about the diet and trying to do it alone
- Failing to pay attention to their vegetable intake
- Focusing on the carbohydrate intake and forgetting about the quality of food
- Drinking too much dairy
- Snacking too much
- Being obsessive about the scale
- Not sleeping enough

How to Recognize Good Fats from Bad Fats

The word 'fat' is something people do not want to be associated with; however, fat plays an integral role in the functioning of the human body. When people hear the word "fat," nothing good comes to their minds, but it is scientifically proven that meals that contain high amounts of fat and low amounts of carbs actually help to reduce weight more effectively than meals that contain low fat.

Fat is an essential element in the human body, and it is impossible to survive without it. However, the problem is that people do not understand the difference between good fats and bad fats. Thus, it is important to understand, and be able to distinguish between good and bad fats, so that people can make the best choices with regards to diets.

What exactly are good fats?

Good fats are mainly saturated fats, unsaturated fats, and trans-fats that exist naturally. In the unsaturated fats category, there are polyunsaturated fats and monounsaturated fats. Good fats contain elements that support heart health and generally lower cholesterol levels in the body, and that is one of the reasons why they should replace all forms of unhealthy saturated fats present in a plethora of diets these days.

It might sound a little bit off-key, but there are zero links between saturated fats and the increase in heart diseases. New studies are starting to change our views on the so-called traditional "bad" fats in our diet.

1.7 Polyunsaturated Fats

Polyunsaturated fats are predominantly found in vegetable oils. They contain elements that help reduce triglyceride and cholesterol levels and are the perfect substitutes for saturated fats. Just like every other thing in life, the keto diet seeks balance, and that's why it is important to maintain a good balance of these fats.

Omega-3 fatty acids are essential to the human body because they contain elements that support heart health, which generally improves human health and sustainability. They are predominantly found in fishes like catfish, mackerel, trout, and salmon, etc. Some plant-based foods that contain these good fats are walnuts and flaxseed.

If you have a deficiency, you can use supplements, but there is nothing better than obtaining your Omega-3 fatty acids from food.

1.8 Monounsaturated Fats

Monounsaturated fats are renowned for their unique ability to mitigate and reduce the risk and impact of heart disease. Mediterranean foods contain a lot of it, and that's because they use a lot of olive oil in the preparation of their dishes. Monounsaturated fats have been credited with the extremely low occurrence of heart diseases in and around the Mediterranean countries. The thing about theses fats is that they become solid when refrigerated, but when stored at room temperature, they maintain their liquid form. When olive oil starts to solidify below 75 degrees Fahrenheit, it points to the fact that you have monounsaturated oil. Vitamin E is another healthy nutrient present in these fats, and it is always better to eat foods that contain these nutrients, as opposed to taking supplements (this is to ensure the best possible effect). Some of the foods that contain these fats include; sesame seeds, nuts, cashew, pumpkin seeds, and olives. Other good sources include peanut oil, canola oil, and olive oil.

Keto and Unsaturated Fats

There are people on the keto diet that make the blunder of consuming huge amounts of fat without much emphasis on the quality, and this is somewhat counterproductive. Thus, it is important to choose your fats correctly because not all fats are the same, and some are far better than others, e.g., fats that emanate from coconut oil and olive oil are good. Also, fats from nuts are good too. While on Keto, it is important always to read nutritional labels to ascertain the type of fats present in your diets; because it will help you stay on course. Finally, it is important to note that most fried foods do not come with enough healthy fats.

Saturated Fat

Over time, it has been said that no matter what happens, people should avoid consuming saturated fats at all costs. However, recent studies have shown that the consumption of saturated fats is in no way associated with greater risks for stroke, heart diseases, and other earlier associated health conditions (and it has nothing to do with gender or age).

Slowly but surely, the perception towards saturated fats is changing, and even the medical community is now getting used to the fact that saturated fats are not as bad as previously thought.

Saturated fats have always been part of human history; for example, coconut oil contains a unique type of saturated fat referred to as medium-chain triglycerides. These fats are extremely easy to digest and transformed into energy.

Since modern research findings have proven that saturated fats are beneficial in healthy dieting, it is now clear that saturated fats are necessary components of a healthy diet.

Saturated Fats and its Health Benefits

Before, the consensus was that saturated fats are completely bad for human health. However, new studies have shown that the position to be wrong and even gone on to show the numerous benefits of saturated fats. In Keto, some of the best sources of saturated fats are cocoa butter, eggs, cream, coconut oil, lard, red meat, and butter, etc. Some of the health benefits include;

Saturated fats help to raise the good blood cholesterol in other to stop the buildup LDL in the arteries.

Saturated fats help in the production of hormones like testosterone and Cortisol. They also help in boosting the immune system to combat infections and diseases.

Saturated fats support bone density, and are also responsible for improved HDL and LDL cholesterol levels.

Natural Trans Fats

Trans fats are mostly bad fats, and it is strange to see them listed in this section. However, the reason they are listed in this section is that there are foods that contain a particular type of "natural" trans-fat. These foods contain trans-fat referred to as Vaccenic acid, and they help maintain heart health, as well as reduce the risk of obesity and diabetes. Healthy trans-fats are mostly found in dairy products and grass-fed meat and are even known to suppress intestinal inflammation and protect against cancer.

What are the bad fats?

For people that intend to lose weight, it is possible to lose weight on the keto diet while consuming bad fats, but there are multiples risks involved. The truth is that you might achieve your primary aim but end up jeopardizing your overall wellbeing, for example, bad fats are known to increase inflammation and are also associated with an increased risk of certain cancer types, including prostate and colon cancer.

The Keto diet is not just about weight loss, and the idea is to live healthy and happy. Thus it is necessary to remove bad fats from your diet completely.

Processed Trans Fats

Not all Trans fats are bad, but the processed ones are as bad as they come. These synthetic fats are bad for human health. Thus it is important to always go for natural Trans fats, as opposed to the processed ones. Most of these processed trans fats are produced from oils made from genetically altered seeds when you consume them, and you are exposed to radical elements that can easily wreak havoc on your body.

Keep away from processed Trans fats.

Dangers of Consuming Trans Fats

There are huge amounts of risks associated with the consumption of processed and adulterated trans-fats, and the likelihood of heart disease is just one of them. People that consume processed foods that contain Trans fats are at a greater risk of developing different forms of cancer. Thus, it is extremely important to consume meats that haven't been processed with chemicals and hormones.

When people consume bad fats, they risk upsetting the equilibrium between good and bad cholesterol levels, which can easily cause inflammation in the body. Furthermore, your gut flora can be destroyed by Trans fats, which also increases the risk of being exposed to all sorts of diseases.

Like I mentioned earlier, there are good and bad trans-fats; you only have to pay close attention in other to figure out which is which. If you come in contact with any type of hydrogenated oil or partially hydrogenated oil, it is important to boycott them. Most times, you'll find them in foods like cookies, margarine, crackers, and some fast food. Some other forms of processed oils you should be on the lookout for include safflower oil, cottonseed oil, canola oil, and sunflower oil. It is important to completely remove these oils from your diet in other to maintain a healthier mind and body.

The Low-Fat Misconception

Most labels on food products come with so much misinformation that it is now difficult to truly ascertain what you're purchasing. It is normal for these companies to withhold names of ingredients and chemicals that were used during production because they believe the quantities are under a certain threshold. Sometimes you'll see labels that read natural and fat-free, but the truth is that they are not always as stated, and some of the added ingredients might even be harmful to human health.

In today's world, there is so much misinformation concerning the types of fat that are safe to consume. However, for people that are on a keto diet, it is important to boycott everything and anything hydrogenated or processed because that is when you'll truly see the effects of a low-carb diet. Don't just buy anything from the mall. Before you do, carefully check the labels and if you find any ingredient you're not familiar with, use the internet to check if it's something you can safely consume.

Finally, one of the things you should lookout for a while checking labels is the length of the ingredients. If you come across an item that has too many ingredients, it is safe to say that you should boycott it, and move on to something with a more streamlined ingredients list.

1.9 Types of Keto Diet

Since the end goal of different variations of the keto diet is the same, these variations share certain similarities, the most notable of which is high dietary fats and low carbohydrates. To put together the right diet, it is important to speak to a doctor or dietician who will give one personalized guidance and advice based on one's individual needs.

Some of the most common types of keto diets include:

1. The common keto diet composed of 20% protein, 70% to 75% fat, and 5% to 10% protein
2. The extremely low carbohydrate keto diet with less than 5% carbohydrate content
3. The well-formulated keto diet with macronutrients of carbohydrates, protein, and fat that meet the requirements or standards of the keto diet
4. The medium-chain triglycerides keto diet
5. Calorie-restricted keto diet
6. Cyclical keto diet
7. Targeted keto diet
8. The high protein keto diet

1.10 Skills for Success in Keto Diet

The keto diet can be extremely difficult to start and maintain since it radically departs from the way people eat these days. The typical American diet, for instance, is high in both processed foods and carbohydrates. The keto diet, however, involves putting the body into a state of ketosis to force it into burning fat for energy.

Some of the skills needed to follow and maintain the keto diet include:

1. Knowing the foods to avoid and eat
2. Understanding one's relationship with fat
3. Improving one's cooking skills
4. Drinking bulletproof coffee, which is one of the best ketogenic-friendly drinks
5. Seeking support from family members and friends

The ketogenic diet or keto, in short, went viral last year. Actually, 2018 was the year of the ketogenic diet. Even today, it shows no signs of slowing down. The internet has tons of guides about this diet because it is somewhat difficult to follow and maintain. There are many different variations of the keto diet plan on the internet. Therefore, it is important to talk to a doctor or dietician before embarking on the ketogenic journey.

Chapter 2: Ketogenic Diet for Women Over 50

After you've had a decent introduction to the keto diet in the first chapter, this chapter will enlighten you on everything you need to know for starting keto as a woman over 50. We'll start with how you can better adapt the diet to your body and particular hormones makeup, which foods to add and what to cut out and what advice you should heed to and what to avoid. Next up, we'll move on to the benefits keto provides for menopausal women with hormonal imbalances, from reducing hot flashes to weight loss to better sleep and so on. We have also included the best low-carb foods for you. Finally, we'll end by discussing the anti-aging benefits of keto.

2.1 How to Adapt To Keto Diet for Women Over 50

Most aspects will continue to change as women mature. The hair and skin will lose their allure, and the new standard is to feel fatigued. You may find an issue, especially throughout your waist, with stomach fat. After a long holiday weekend in the past, it may have been easy to lose a pound or two, but now you're trapped all year with the excess weight. It is statistically known that males usually lose weight more easily than females. It's attributed to body structure and testosterone. Even so, if women make several adjustments to the ketogenic diet schedule, they will shed body fat effectively, thus feel and look refreshed as well.

1. Slowly Reduce Your Carb Intake

Typically, switching from the normal 330g of carbohydrates per day to 25g is not an issue for men. Reducing carb consumption drastically throws the metabolism of the body towards ketosis, and that's when accumulated fat is consumed. Although women can effectively reduce the number of carbohydrates they eat, for sustainability, they have to do so at a gradual rate than men.

Dietitians suggest that women steadily reduce carbohydrates across a few weeks to ensure that their hormones remain balanced. For the first week, start with about 150g and afterward drop to 100g during the next week. The body will have adapted to 25g of carbs a day within a month.

In general, a drop in glucose levels, a rise in triglyceride levels, and a reduction of 19 pounds were found in women who used this procedure and remained at 25g of carbohydrates per day for two months. The effects on your body moving through ketosis vary from person to person, but that is an excellent technique.

2. Don't Try To Reduce Calories

Note, unintentional calorie control is a big advantage in keto. By limiting them more, don't try to overdo it. If this isn't what you believe in, give it three weeks. Three weeks of consuming ad-libitum. Don't get stuffed. Don't fill your coffee with a pound of butter simply because you're now on keto. But don't calorie-count. Don't calculate and check too much.

Feed till you feel full. Feed till you are no longer hungry. Don't eat till you're stuffed. You get a lot of room between "under-eating" and "stuffing." Most people who consume a simple keto diet of whole foods would not have difficulty remaining between the lines. Know that your unconscious mechanisms can regulate the ingestion of calories for you. Don't cheat the body; allow it the opportunity to run.

3. Do Fasting or Keto: Choose One

Also, certain males, who appear to be more resilient to metabolic diseases, suffer from intensive fasting or continuously shortened feeding windows while mixing exceedingly low-carb diets. Their calorie intake is going too low for too long, too rapidly. The aim of low carb diets is to maximize fat oxidation. The aim of fasting is to maximize the burning of fat. They are shooting for really similar stuff when you conclude it. Integrating the two sounds that the rewards will be supercharged. But that may not be the case, especially for a woman, especially when you start your diet first. Besides, it becomes impossible to decide what is causing the damage (or advantage) if you perform all of them in one go. Introduce one big change at a time to allow yourself a better understanding of the condition. Fast or do keto, not both.

4. Don't Avoid fat in the Beginning

Furthermore, it will mean that you will not have a calorie deficit working on you. This gives the body a warning of waste, which means that it will not dive into the metabolic defensive style and stick for life to stored fat.

In addition, it provides you with emotional assistance. It's a good way to note that more fat can be eaten than you think would be advantageous and still lose fat and have medicinal benefits. It also tends to break down the psychological block that everybody has when eating fat because of having grown up in a low-fat age. Giving yourself permission to eat a lot (maybe even too much) of fat at the Beginning pushes the pendulum squarely in the opposite way so that it can land comfortably in the middle where it originally belonged.

Except if you're looking to add weight, this huge fat spike does not linger. If you get better at generating and absorbing ketones and, gradually, fat mass, you can begin consuming away at your adipose tissues and lowering the amount of dietary fat. Maintaining the extra fat intake, though, maybe appropriate for those who are undernourished or who use keto clinically. Nevertheless, this might go for all of us: if you've been eating a low-fat diet for so long, a seeming "big boost" in fat intake will only help you achieve what can be considered normal ketone levels.

5. Be Wary of Keto Snacks

For Keto sportsmen who require as many extra calories enough to sustain metabolism, fat bombs may be useful buddies. Because of the sheer amount of food they consume, these folks typically attain sufficient micro-nutrition. Do not copy anything if it doesn't fit you. The healthiest options are:

- Pork rinds
- Couple oz. of cheese
- Avocado egg salad
- Olives
- Nut butter on celery sticks (add salt if unsalted)
- Collagen smoothies
- Egg yolks
- Veggie-loaded guacamole: avocados, salt, lime, peppers, herbs, tomatoes, garlic
- Avocados, avocados chopped up with sardines
- Boiled eggs

6. Don't Be So Hard On Yourself

In the Beginning, there's a case for extreme stringency. During the initial month, staying as precisely as possible with keto works great for your system to get used to switching fuel resources. So you're fine until you're there. The system is made to burn fat. The cells are excellent at alternating between sugar and fat. Your child delighted you by presenting a delicious gluten-free treat that is not likely to wreck your whole keto path. You're bound to recover fully. You're going to be great.

If you are attempting to avert epileptic fits, boost the impact of chemotherapy medications, cure Parkinson's disease, or, for some other identifiable condition, require strong ketone levels, remain strict. Don't be too strict, otherwise.

7. Don't Follow the Traditional Advice Too Keenly

If the diet "does not succeed," which, of course, typically implies that the individual does not lose weight, you hear 3 things:

- Reduce your calories
- Reduce your protein
- Reduce carbohydrates to 20g

But, less is not always the solution for a system that is under pressure. Often the body wants more to consume, maybe more carbohydrates or proteins in particular. With IF and severe calorie counting, people typically move right from the Standard American Diet, or also from higher-carb paleo directly into rigid keto all in one big go. Your body requires time to understand how to fuel itself with ketones, so it can be completely problematic to strip away all nutritional protection at the very same time. And since women are generally more susceptible than men to metabolic abnormalities or starvation signs, they especially need to listen to this advice.

8. Don't Restrict Protein Too Much

A menopausal woman goes on the keto and gets bad results. She uses the internet, questions, and they reply, "Go low on protein." She lowers protein and produces bad outcomes. Then she decreases her protein a little further, and she struggles further. She soon consumes nothing but mayo from the kitchen, nuts and some baby spinach. She's on keto, and somehow her problems are still steadily becoming worse.

True, too much protein is capable of impairing ketogenesis. Individuals whose wellness necessitates elevated amounts of systemic ketones must reduce protein, believe it or not. And, in the traditional diets for epilepsy, there isn't enough protein. Protein consumption is still too poor, particularly for the average female citizen who already prefer to consume lesser protein than males. If you lack lean muscle, continue to lag in the workout, and having worse body structure changes, receiving elevated ketone levels is not worth much.

9. Cut Out Alcohol

Many individuals enjoy the idea that they may have a bottle of dry wine from moment to moment on a low-carb or keto diet. If you are feeling a plateau in weight loss or adding weight, though, cut out all alcohol as of now before weight loss begins again. A drink or two a week could also trigger a pause.

10. Avoid Artificial Sweeteners

The experts advise to wean yourself off them if you have used chemical sweeteners such as sucralose or aspartame in your low carb diet. Although there's not a number of research trials, experts find from anecdotal experience that as individuals get rid of synthetic sweeteners, they will lose weight.

2.2 Benefits of Keto Diet For Menopause And Hormonal Imbalances

Menopause typically starts between the ages of 45 and 55 and is characterized by the discontinuation of the menstrual period of a woman. This adjustment phase will last anything between seven to 14 years, and signs, including hot flashes and shifts of mood, sometimes occur. There are also metabolic variations in certain women that can contribute to obesity and, in some situations, insulin resistance.

Menopause is a normal progression of physiology that all females go through. This change may, nevertheless, be difficult for certain females.

With variations in estrogen and progesterone (the hormone levels responsible for monitoring one's menstrual periods), your body may start behaving irregularly, and it can create a series of chronic stress.

Menopause usually happens gradually. Currently, in your 30's, the gradual and normal loss of estrogen and progesterone starts.

Many of the typical symptoms encountered by peri-menopausal and post-menopausal women include:

- Sleep problems

- Slowed metabolism
- Thinning hair
- Brain fog
- Mood changes
- Night sweats
- Hot flashes
- Vaginal dryness
- Cravings
- Irregular periods

Fortunately, there is no reason for this normal phase to be as unpleasant as it sounds. Monitoring your lifestyle will have a substantial influence on how your body progresses during menopause. Excess weight and insulin resistance are two menopause signs that are specifically linked with food and lifestyle.

Simply changing your food is a straightforward technique under the supervision of a health professional that will better stabilize your estrogen levels and relieve some menopause symptoms. Apparently, low-carb, high-fat diets are trending a bunch. It receives a tremendous amount of respect from people of diverse cultures since it promotes their well-being and lifestyle. The keto diet is, in particular, a high-fat, relatively low-carb diet that is sometimes prescribed to alleviate the effects of menopause. So, we'll look at how the ketogenic diet helps with the effects of menopause in this section.

1. Weight Loss

Data suggests that as opposed to the vegan diet or a low-fat diet, a low-carb diet is a better option for maintaining weight after menopause.

There are many variables that may lead to the advantages of low-carb eating throughout menopause for weight loss.

One is the effect on muscle mass that low-carb, ketogenic diets provide. It is possible that adopting some weight reduction regimen would contribute to a degree of muscle loss. This is attributed to the reality that certain muscles naturally go along for the ride while you burn fat.

In an attempt to lose bodyweight, often, people who go through menopause pursue tactics such as calorie control or low-fat diets. The drawback to these diet strategies is that they sometimes result in considerable levels of muscle reduction, further exhausting your metabolic rate.

While there is no dispute that physical exercise is needed to preserve muscle and good body structure, there is some indication that low-carb eating can have a more muscle-saving impact than any other diet for weight loss.

The impact that low-carb eating has on insulin regulation is another aspect. Data indicates that eating a low-carbohydrate diet not only leads to a reduced intake of energy but it also affects insulin sensitivity, resulting in improved regulation of blood glucose.

One research also showed that in post-menopausal women, three low-carb square meals in 24 hours resulted in a 30 percent drop in insulin resistance. Furthermore, the subjects developed elevated fasting insulin release and insulin resistance when subjects were offered high-carb foods for 5 days.

The reduction of appetite, which may be predicted to push down ghrelin levels to some degree, is a major benefit of being in ketosis. A Keto Diet helps to balance out leptin hormones that induce appetite and wipes off urges so that you can get smaller and improve your fitness. A low-carb, nutrient-rich, paleo diet allows the abdomen and visceral fat to decline more dramatically and triglyceride levels to fall.

2. Mood Swings

Mood control is one of the functions that estrogen performs in the body. That is why, during your menstrual period, you may encounter highs and lows in your mood. For certain females, the initiation of menopause is followed by depression because of the function of estrogen in the control of neurotransmitters.

Research indicates that via multiple mechanisms, namely neurotransmitter control, mitochondrial activity, and the modulation of oxidative damage, the ketogenic diet may affect mood. Studies also claim that the ketogenic diet has an antidepressant impact due to its mood-improving function.

3. Energy

For women who are undergoing menopause, tiredness and nausea are two typical symptoms. It makes sense that your whole hormone structure is transforming, and your body is going through a new period of existence that will certainly zap your resources. This will set someone up for exhaustion, coupled with the shifts in glucose metabolism that come with decreasing amounts of estrogen.

However, you're no more at the mercy of caffeine when it tends to come to calories as you adopt a keto diet. The primary distinction between carbohydrates as energy and ketones as energy is that insulin is necessary for glucose to control it and sustain steady blood glucose levels.

On the other end, ketones are in ample abundance. Ketone development is a stable operation, unlike the spikes that you experience with blood sugar. Conclusion? Throughout the day, the vitality is maintained, ensuring that the wall you normally encounter at about 2 pm is a distant memory.

When transitioning to a ketogenic diet, most females are going through menopause report amazing quantities of energy. This is when your sugar levels return to normal, and your blood sugars no longer see drastic peaks and drops. The keto diet is indeed unbelievably time-efficient. A fasting portion is part of the ketogenic diet, mostly intermittent fasting, that is when you can comfortably manage 13 to 15 hours each day without food.

If you're like a lot of people who are menopausal, you have such a mad stressful schedule. Careers, commute, social needs, taking children to athletic activities, meeting children of college-age, etc. If you introduce the keto diet, from carbohydrate consumption to fat burning, you change the energy supply. This suggests that you will go without eating for lengthy stretches of time. For the overstressed racing menopausal lady, there is nothing more comfortable than not needing to feed every several hours. Often, fasting is an excellent way to refresh the microbiota.

4. The Cravings

When they go into menopause, often, females develop sweet cravings. It can be for delicious, high-carb items such as cookies or pies or sausage and French fries for savory, fatty foods. Either case, these eating habits will lead to complications such as weight gain and exhaustion and intensify the menopause's often painful symptoms.

The impact on cravings is one of the first advantages that individuals report during a ketogenic diet. When adopting a keto diet, the mid-afternoon hanger tends to vanish entirely, and the sweet tooth becomes a distant memory.

This is possibly due to keto's blood-sugar controlling influence. You don't have the regular ups and downs of energy that contribute to food cravings because the body depends on glucose for nutrition. One research found that adopting a ketogenic diet culminated in a substantial decrease in cravings, coupled with healthier sleep and an enhanced sense of well-being, and an increased feeling of satiety. Given that emotional conflict is one of the key factors for bingeing, this suggests that on many occasions, keto may help curb your cravings.

5. Cures Insulin Resistance

Menopause will reduce the adequacy of insulin, which will impair the capacity of the body to properly utilize insulin. Insulin, as well as other hormones, is regulated by the keto diet, meaning you suffer less adverse effects, including hair loss and night sweats. Also, if they do arise, they are relatively shorter and not uncomfortable. As per the studies, to control blood glucose levels more effectively, a keto diet can treat insulin resistance. One research showed that in women with the endometrial or ovarian lesion, after a ketogenic diet for around three months, insulin sensitivity increased.

Reducing carb-dependence will decrease the amounts of insulin and increase the unbalanced condition of hormones, resulting in beneficial effects during menopause.

6. Reduced Hot Flashes And Night Sweats

Many women beginning a keto diet experience less serious and rare hot flashes and night sweats. In a few instances, the change is swift and lasting by both reports. Brain function drops at the stage that glucose does not reach into the brain, causing a rise in hot flashes. This form is much about what occurs with epilepsy in young boys, while menopausal ladies undergo it to a much smaller degree. One of the tasks of estrogen is to bring glucose from food into your cerebrum, so as estrogen decreases after menopause, so does the ability to get sugar into your head. A diet focused on keto cleans out this glucose issue, reducing the frequency and severity of hot flashes in women with symptoms of menopause. By maintaining an incredibly low-carb diet that supplies the brain with ketone bodies, which it can use for power, those who suffer the adverse effects of hot flashes can limit their recurrence and intensity.

7. Improved libido

Ever-fluctuating hormones, loss of confidence and libido can be one menopause symptom. A high-fat diet regimen, though, can help balance out all levels of estrogen and testosterone, thereby contributing to boost libido. A Keto diet rich in sound fat improves the preservation of fat-solvent nutrients, especially nutrient D, a precursor to your sex hormones. A regimen of eating focused on keto helps regulate testosterone and other hormones, which are completely messed up owing to menopause, thereby improving sex life.

8. Improved Sleeping Patterns

High amounts of sugar and processed carbs are correlated with a low standard of sleep. It seems like the essence and origins of carbs seemed to be a greater concern than their size. The disparity between those who consume a lot of carbs and get disrupted sleep each night is in the former eating refined baked goods and outdoor foods than others who get quality rest with a comparable amount of carb consumption. Numerous people mention resting even more deeply on the keto diet than people who have never done a ketogenic diet in the first place.

9. Reduced Inflammation

During menopause, never-ending inflammation will intensify, causing serious symptoms and taking a crucial place in essentially every disease on this planet. A nutritional routine focused on keto consolidates anti-inflammatory fats with antacid-rich nutrients, reducing joint pain, back pain, and other such disorders.

Keto Diet and Hormonal Imbalance

In our environment, hormonal irregularities are highly common and may lead to several various health conditions. By enhancing insulin efficiency, a Keto diet will potentially assist with hormonal problems. Insulin resistance is increasingly widespread today, but before they experience severe chronic health conditions, most individuals remain unaware of the concern. Cortisol is also influenced by this diet plan. A hormone produced by the adrenal glands is cortisol. Sitting over your kidneys, they secrete chemicals into the circulatory system and react to input from several other chemicals and hormones in your system as well. As we consume carbs (causing the blood sugar to increase too fast and drop easily, causing a stress reaction), and gradually they become unable to restore themselves, you will induce adrenal fatigue by placing strain on your adrenal glands from a sugar response.

Ultimately, relative to carbohydrate diets, ketogenic foods, such as keto bars, are less stressful on the body, which may help enhance the control of cortisol metabolism. It will also help encourage your hormones to regain their equilibrium again by restricting the level of sugar in the blood, thus decreasing your insulin resistance. PCOS, which impacts 1 in 10 females, is a widespread condition induced by hormonal imbalances in women.

Best Low-Carb Foods for Menopause

Continuing to follow a keto diet implies that there is a back-burner for items such as bread and potatoes, whereas high-quality protein and fats are essential to the diet. Generally speaking, cutting down on carbohydrates and adding additional fat into the diet is an ideal way to treat menopause.

However, because of their balanced fat and vitamin quality, there are also several low-carbohydrate diets that are particularly helpful for females undergoing menopause. Focus on foods rich in omega-3 fatty acids, calcium, and fiber, including the following examples:

- Grass-fed beef
- Broccoli
- Kale
- Full-fat dairy (cheese, milk, yogurt)
- Sunflower seeds
- Sesame seeds
- Fatty fish (salmon, mackerel)
- Flax seeds

Women's well-being will, at times, sound like a shifting goal. It is no surprise why so many people feel exhausted, depleted, and overweight because of the ever-fluctuating amounts of female hormones and chemical problems that can arise during the lifespan. And as you begin having menopausal symptoms, this appears twice as apparent.

Luckily, when stuff seems out of whack, Mother Nature always has a solution. During this critical period of transformation, the health benefits of maintaining a high-fat diet whilst in a ketosis state could be really be all you need to feel at your best.

2.3 Anti-Ageing Benefits of Keto Diet

Low-carb diets are by far the most famous for the purposes of losing weight. How it will delay the aging process and keep you fresh and healthy is a less-understood but maybe more meaningful advantage of a low-carb diet. It also has to do about how the restriction of carbohydrates will reduce blood glucose and insulin, which has an anti-aging impact in response.

You are more susceptible to undergo surges and drops of blood sugar as you intake a significant percentage of your food from processed carbohydrates and sugar. This nutritional pattern, along with an absence of physical training, promotes weight gain while also contributing to higher levels of insulin.

You already recognize that the pancreas produces insulin to enable the body to consume it for fuel or preserve the glucose for future use as fat. This all happens after a meal. Blood sugar may be dangerous and can lead to coma, and even mortality, at significantly elevated levels. The pancreas, thus, seeks to balance blood glucose levels firmly. The body seems to do a decent job of controlling sugar levels when we consume a nutritious diet of natural foods such as that of our predecessors (meat, seafood, veggies, fruits, nuts, seeds).

When our meals are rich in processed carbs, fructose, as well as other packaged foods, the body doesn't work too well. Sugar levels increase very quickly in reaction to the standard American diet, and it is normal for the pancreas to misjudge the dose of insulin required to get sugar levels down to a healthy level. Cells grow less sensitive to insulin over time, and much more is required, causing a steady decline of insulin response and high levels of blood sugar.

High blood glucose levels motivate the body to create complex proteins known as AGEs (a term for advanced glycation end-products). Glycation is darkening in simplistic words, like the darkening that happens whenever you slice an apple in two and leave it to rest. In this situation, the oxygen interacts with the proteins in the apple to induce oxidation and color alteration.

AGEs behave the same as free radicals, floating freely and causing damage to cells and DNA. They build up and trigger wrinkles and harm to the blood vessels in the skin. In the occurrence of chronic conditions, such as coronary failure, Alzheimer's, and metabolic disorders, AGEs are also involved.

One method of counteracting this is a low-carb lifestyle. Studies have repeatedly demonstrated that a low-carb diet can decrease sugar and blood insulin levels, decrease glycation, and the number of AGEs that injure tissues and organs in a range of populations like those with obesity or diabetes.

As one of the key causes of premature aging, the Free Radical Theory of Aging relates to oxidative stress. If there are not enough antioxidants to battle off free radicals in our cells, oxidative stress arises. Free radicals are lacking an electron, so they are trying to "snatch" electrons from other molecules that have a cascade effect that contributes to cell damage. So, to avoid this, it's necessary for the body to have healthy antioxidants.

In each cell, mitochondria play an essential role. It is essential for energy output and the control of mitochondrial function. There is a reduction in the efficiency and function of the mitochondria as we mature. One research indicates that mitochondrial glutathione amounts are boosted by this diet plan. One of the only antioxidants which can find a way into the mitochondria is glutathione.

2.4 Other Benefits of Keto Diet

The keto diet is one of the most popular diets today, which is why there are more than a million Google searches every month for this diet. Some of the reasons for its popularity include:

1. It Helps People Lose Weight

Initially, weight loss results from loss of water because of the drastic reduction in carbohydrate intake. The keto diet also encourages people to consume foods rich in fat and cut back on carbohydrates, sugar, and refined carbohydrates. This will lead to a constant supply of energy and fewer sugar highs and crashes.

Actually, the first thing people on this diet report is having steady energy and not needing to snack all the time due to waning energy. Essentially, the keto diet often lowers the desire to eat and leads to fewer hunger pangs. If one is not hungry all the time, one will eat less, which will lead to weight loss.

Interestingly, although the keto diet is high in fat content, it is often more effective when it comes to helping people lose weight than a low-fat diet. However, it is not right for everyone. While it may lead to short-term weight loss, it is extremely difficult to follow.

2. Treating Epilepsy in Kids

The only clear and proven health benefit of the keto diet is its ability to reduce epileptic seizures in kids. In fact, since 1920, doctors have been using it therapeutically for this very purpose. Experts recommend the keto diet for children suffering from certain conditions, such as Rett syndrome or Lennox-Gastaut syndrome, and do not respond to medication for seizure.

The Epilepsy Foundation suggests that the ketogenic diet can decrease the number of seizures kids have by up to 50%, with about 10% to 15% of children becoming seizure-free. The foundation also notes that this diet can also be beneficial for adults who suffer from epilepsy, although it is quite difficult and restrictive to stick with.

3. May Improve Heart Health

When a person follows the keto diet in a healthy manner, it can improve the health of his/her heart by reducing bad cholesterol. In addition, this diet also increases the levels of HDL-cholesterol, which is good cholesterol.

4. Reduces Acne

There are many different forms of acne, and some may have a connection to blood sugar and diet. A diet rich in refined and processed carbohydrates, for example, can alter the bacteria in the gut and dramatic fluctuations in the levels of blood sugar, which can have a negative effect on skin health. Limiting carbohydrates intake; therefore, can help reduce some forms of acne.

5. Metabolic Syndrome

Limited research suggests that adults suffering from the metabolic disease can benefit from the keto diet because it can help them get rid of more body fat and weight, compared to people who eat a diet heavy in added sugars and processed foods.

6. Type 2 Diabetes

In September 2016, the Journal of Obesity and Eating Disorders published research suggesting that the keto diet could be helpful to people with type-2 diabetes and lead to improvements in the levels of HbA1c. However, it is important to understand that it can also lead to low blood sugar levels, also called hypoglycemia, if the patient also takes medication to lower his/her blood sugar.

7. Bipolar Disorder

The keto diet may be a mood stabilizer for individuals with type 2 bipolar disorder. According to a study published in the journal Neurocase in October 2012, in certain cases, it may be more effective than medication.

8. Obesity

According to one study published in the journal Endocrine in December 2016, obese people on a low-calorie keto diet lose ore inflammatory belly fat as compared to those on a normal low-calorie diet. In addition, according to a February 2018 article published in the journal Nutrition and Metabolism, this diet may also help maintain a lean body mass during weight loss.

9. Alzheimer's Disease and Dementia

An article in the journal Neurobiology of Aging published in February 2013 suggested that higher-risk older adults on a ketogenic diet experienced significantly better memory functioning after one and a half months.

Certain experts in the field of Alzheimer's, such as the director of the Alzheimer's Prevention Clinic at Weill Cornell Medicine and New York Presbyterian, Richard Issacson, MD, suggest low-carbohydrate diets as one of the ways to delay brain aging, and maybe even Alzheimer's, which is a form of dementia.

10. Parkinson's Disease

Since people with this condition tend to have a higher risk of developing dementia, experts like Robert Krikorian, Ph.D., a professor of clinical psychiatry, are conducting studies looking at whether inducing dietary ketosis can preserve cognitive functioning. Only time and more research will tell.

11. Certain Forms of Cancer

Some studies, such as one published in the journal Oncology in November 2018; suggest that doctors should use the ketogenic diet in conjunction with radiation and chemotherapy to treat certain forms of cancer.

However, to determine whether this diet can play a helpful role in cancer therapy, scientists need to conduct more studies. More importantly, without a doctor's consent, patients should not use the keto diet as a stand-alone treatment for any disease.

12. Polycystic Ovary Syndrome

Women with this infertility condition have a higher risk of developing obesity and diabetes. This is why some medical professionals recommend the ketogenic diet. However, researchers need to conduct long-term research on the safety of using the keto diet to deal with this condition.

- **Other Unexpected Benefits**

Some researchers suggest the possibility of gaining several other unexpected benefits from the keto diet. These findings, however, are preliminary and require more research. These include:

1. The diminishment of anxiety and depression
2. A healthier liver
3. A fall in inflammation markers
4. Sound sleep

Chapter 3: Getting Started With Keto

In this chapter, we are going to talk about how you can start your keto diet journey after eating poorly all your life. We will also take a look at the ways in which you can recognize how unhealthily you've been eating by looking at all the signs your body has been sending you all along that you totally ignored. Lastly, we'll shed light on some tips and tricks on what you can do about your poor eating to change for the better.

3.1 How to Start Keto After Years of Poor Eating Habits?

A high-fat and very low carb diet plan, the ketogenic diet, maybe challenging to initiate. After all, that is definitely a dramatic deviation from the way you consume food now (carbohydrates and refined foods are heavy in a conventional American diet. If you're trying low-carb, high-fat eating, evade problems and set yourself up for a successful weight loss, here are the steps you need to take to start a keto diet after years of poor eating habits.

1. Know What to Eat and Avoid

You'll severely restrict carbohydrates by implementing a keto diet program. Begin with 20 to 30 g of carbs a day. Be sure you already know what foods mainly comprise of sugars, fat, and protein, so you can make good choices. It's not only foods like pizza, spaghetti, cookies, chips, and hot chocolate that have carbohydrates, for starters. Beans can have protein, but they are really rich in carbs as well. Carbs are often present in berries and plants. Meat (protein) and natural fats such as oil and butter (such as olive oil and coconut oil) are the other items that do not include carbs.

2. Fix Your Relationship with Fat

People fear fat as they've been warned it's going to kill them. What's frustrating is that today's science appears contradictory. Some research indicates that it is important to substitute saturated fat with unsaturated fats (and eliminate dangerous trans fats) to reduce the risk of cardiac attack, although others suggest that cardiovascular issues have not been linked with overall fat and forms of fat. It gets complicated to know how precisely to consume them. It is also helpful to note that food is more than just a fixed ingredient, and therefore it counts for the overall consistency of the diet. Start making minor changes to what you consume every day to brace for a high-fat diet, which may feel unpleasant at first, such as ordering a sandwich on lettuce and substituting leafy greens for fries.

3. Change How You See Protein

Most of the low carb diet and lifestyle's more popular myths is that you can consume as much protein as you'd like. But it isn't a plan where you only focus on carbs. You will need to keep the consumption of protein reasonable. It is possible to convert protein into glucose, so bingeing on protein will take the system out of ketogenic mode. Think of the proportions as a tiny meat section blanketed with a substantial quantity of fat.

4. Learn To Cook

For keto-approved dishes you'll enjoy, look at a number of keto blogs and cookbooks. Experts consider selecting four or five food recipes that you believe you're going to enjoy. You don't hang around the way, deciding what and what not to eat, then resort to carbs.

5. Try Bulletproof Coffee

This beverage will help hold your appetite at bay by adding coconut oil and butter into the coffee, allowing you time to prepare your next meal. Just remember that coconut oil has the ability to raise bad cholesterol levels, so you certainly would like to limit this drink if you have heart problems or are at higher risk for it because of your personal and family health records.

6. Talk to Your Family

The best aspect of making a major improvement in the food you eat is often coping with the responses of other people. At better, they might doubt your decision; at the very worst, with a container filled with starchy foods, they may show up at the door. If somebody is attempting to undermine your great attempts with a sentence of your choosing, practice respectfully refusing. Consider saying things like, "I am pleased about what I consume," or "Right now, I'm sorting out what feels right for my health."

Notify them regarding your strategy. During family dinners, you will not be willing to consume what they're consuming, so you'll like to prep them (and one) for what your new eating habits may look like. As this plan is mostly only carried out for a brief period (3 to 6 months), you should tell them that it is brief.

7. Up Your Electrolytes

The kidneys release extra electrolytes during ketosis. Focus on getting the potassium and sodium your system requires to operate well. Salt the food, drink salted chicken soup, and consume Brussel sprouts, broccoli, bell peppers, and baby spinach for non-starchy vegetables.

3.2 Ways to Identify Poor Eating Habits?

It's not just your midsection that can let you know if your eating is in need of an upgrade. Sure, the need to reconsider what you introduce into your body may be indicated by weight gain. However, research still suggests that certain such medical issues are involved in unhealthy eating patterns.

The correct nutrients in the correct dosage are the secret to a healthy and stable lifespan, and when you grow older, the requirements of your body adjust. You don't need as many calories; for example, however, you require more minerals, such as levels of vitamin D. And your body could have difficulty taking in and utilizing vitamins contained in foods, such when B12, as you mature. Older people don't often have the foods they need due to this.

Usually, these symptoms do not appear suddenly, but with time, they start to appear.

1. You're Gassy All the Time

Among the most prevalent signs of a poor diet is gas. This also happens because of the fact that the foods you consume do not react well to the bacteria in the digestive tract, resulting in discomfort and flatulence. Surplus gas may be a rationale for modifying the diet: in case of allergies, try leaving out gluten-containing or dairy ingredients or minimizing the intake of carbonated drinks since they have been documented to produce excess gas.

A big sign of a poor diet is persistent bloat. You may be allergic to milk if you find that you're frequently puffy and gassy after consuming dairy or cheese. Numerous people are slightly intolerant of milk but don't even know it, just remember to read the indications that your body gives you.

2. Your Hair Is Like Straw

In order to work properly, the organs need sufficient nutrients, and safe hair cells are no different. Starvation diets may cause fragile hair, or even worse, baldness, contributing to extreme malnutrition. Studies suggest that hair loss, thinning hair and paleness of skin tone are correlated with intakes that are deficient in calcium, important essential fats, and vitamins and minerals like vitamin C, iron and zinc. For good hair, reach for lean protein sources (think poultry and grilled fish), lots of vegetables and fruits, and nuts and seeds.

3. Premature Aging

Aging is unavoidable. But an emerging body of literature shows that a healthy diet can improve the wellbeing of the skin and suppress external symptoms of skin aging. A 2012 prospective study found that, in addition to main flavonoids and antioxidants, a diet high in vitamin A, C, D and E have favorable effects on the skin. Eat five or six servings per day of fruits and vegetables in order to get the rewards and a much more vibrant look.

4. Dental And Gum Problems

Our mouth is one of the first sites that will exhibit signs of an inadequate diet. Bleeding, sore gums may trigger gum disease due to a deficiency of vitamin C. You might also lose some teeth in extreme situations. It may alter your dietary habits if you do have dental implants or lost or weak teeth. A bad diet is, therefore, a double-edged sword: It is much difficult to consume nutritious meals if your gum hurts, and you have trouble with your mouth. And that renders maintaining your teeth protected tougher.

Teeth and gums that are agitated or swollen are both indicators of poor eating habits. A reason for cavities is so much sugar. Consider how much sugary beverages and snacks you eat whenever you end up at the dental professional for fillers. Furthermore, sore or infected gums are also related to too little vitamin C in the diet. With foods such as bananas, broccoli, green leafy vegetables and potato, you can improve your vitamin C.

5. Excessive Weight Gain / Loss

A typical warning sign of bad eating habits is unintended weight gain or loss. Unintended weight loss, especially in disease-related situations, tends to be a major predictor of malnutrition. Typically, unintended excess weight means that the diet is high with refined carbohydrates that put on weight but supply your body with no nutritious benefit. It is necessary to up your intake of healthy foods that bring in fiber and healthy protein to help control weight. Chickpeas, tofu, chickpeas, and popcorn provide few decent and healthy alternatives.

6. Brain Activity Depleted

Popular warning signs of inadequate dietary consumption are identified by problems with recollection and/or focus. To stay stable and work correctly, the human brain relies on a sufficient diet, primarily an appropriate supply of essential fatty acids. The role of omega 3 fatty acids in brain development at any and all stages of life has been highlighted by several researchers. By selecting foods rich in omega-3 fatty acids like walnuts, fish oil, flaxseed and wild salmon, integrate lots of DHA into the eating habits.

7. Digestive Issues

Hard stools and other infrequent bowel movement patterns are a telling sign of something that is flawed in your food intake. You definitely do not have sufficient fiber in your diet if you have constipation problems. The gastrointestinal system is regulated by fiber, and it all goes fine, so eating a healthy diet with loads of fiber is vital. Good sources of fiber include foods, including beans, peas, and whole grains.

The quickest indication that you have a poor dietary consumption of fiber, especially soluble fiber, will also be intestinal distress. As a consequence of insufficient intake of fiber, both indigestion and diarrhea can emerge. Research has shown that soluble fiber has the potential to prolong stomach emptying, which enhances sensations of satiation, improves nutrient absorption in the small bowel, and encourages adequate stool development.

8. You're Always Hungry

You keep convincing yourself you're about to go on a detox, but you're breaking and enjoying a whole chocolate bar and a bowl of frozen yogurt at the close of the day. While your motivation has much to do with this, the source of the issue could also be your diet. Binge eating is the manner your body responds to not receiving the nutrition you need. It's a physiological reaction and a mind warning that you don't offer it what it wants.

You may assume you're only hungry because the food you have eaten has been digested by your body, and it wants to get more nutrition, but your appetite may simply be the product of not getting the right kinds of nutrition for your food. Foods high in sugar or salt, quick carbs, and soda, for instance, might persuade you that you are complete-a hamburger with fries and a beverage looks like a full meal, but the body can digest them much faster, leading you to hunger faster. As a consequence, you are expected to consume full meals a day and consume more often than if you were consuming nutrient-dense, protein-filled meats, complex carbs, and good fats.

9. Bad Skin

Although you will assume that when you complete adolescence, the face zits will end, you may notice that flare-ups will result from bad nutrition. As vitamin A plays an essential part in maintaining the skin clean and stable, this may be attributed to malnutrition. Candies and carbohydrates, greasy goods, and animal items include other perpetrators for inducing acne on the face.

10. Memory Problems

This can have a detrimental impact on many body functions, whether you are not getting enough nutrition or consuming a low-calorie diet. This might render details, like details for an entrance interview, very challenging to recall.

And the items you consume influence your recollection. Women who eat more saturated fats ranked poorly on recall and thought measures relative to those who skipped these foods, according to a report by Annals of Neurology. By dumping the junk food and fries and opting for anything with no saturated fat, like kale or an avocado toast, keep your memory fresh.

11. Ridged or Spoon-Shaped Nails

A bad diet may trigger the nail to alter many times. Your nails can become dry and fragile, much like your skin, but there could also be other indicators. One is nails, particularly on the index finger or the ring finger; they will curve like a tsp. This can mean that you are short on iron. Also, the nails can be ridged or tend to fall away from the nail bed. Nail issues may be triggered by insufficient protein, calcium, or vitamin A, B6, C, and D intakes, in addition to iron problems.

12. You're Always in a Bad Mood

Your food could be destroying your happiness if you're constantly grumpy. You'll get annoyed with cravings as you cut down on sugar and refined carbs. And your sugar levels are still poor, as per doctors, which leads to mood fluctuations. Experts consider introducing more carbohydrates to your foods, which can make you full for longer and would also help your brain generate serotonin (the "happiness" chemical).

13. You're Constantly Cold

In season, if you require a coat, the odds are that your food is off-balanced. The research reported in the Journal of the American College of Nutrition reveals that a low-carb diet will have a detrimental impact on your thyroid, which influences the temperature of the body. A sluggish thyroid can make you feel cold all the time. Instead of cutting all carbohydrates, make sure you consume healthy stuff that comes from whole grain stuff, pasta, and other baked goods.

14. You're Depressed

When you've been feeling miserable, the cause might be something you eat on a regular basis. The Indian Psychiatry Journal reported that vitamin, mineral, and/ or omega-3 fats deficit would potentially contribute to depression and other psychiatric illnesses. They also noticed that taking antioxidants and vitamin B12 dietary supplements helped patients improve their morale and counter their psychiatric disorders.

15. Fatigue

One of the main measures of the standard of the food may be energy levels. If you're dealing with chronically low amounts of energy, your food is likely to be high on carbs and short on protein. Studies suggest that mixing lean protein with whole grains will help balance your blood glucose levels and help raise your levels of energy. Your consumption of vitamin C could also be on the lesser-side. As an afternoon pick-me-up, a report suggests Vitamin C.

3.3 Tips to Avoid Poor Eating Habits

We're just creatures of habit. From the very same grocery shop, we buy the same items, cook the same meals over and over again and function inside our own comfortable habits. Yet you ought to mix things up, alter your unhealthy eating patterns, and begin to think more about your food and lifestyle if you're concerned about eating healthy and weight loss. The thing is, in certain ways, we get so relaxed that it is impossible to give up some old patterns.

Many individuals are reluctant to modify their lifestyles since they have gotten used to consuming or consuming the same meals, so there is an apprehension of the unexpected or doing something different. So, no matter how diligent you can be with your sleep routine or getting in some morning exercises on your weight-loss mission, there is no ignoring the reality that you have kept a few unhealthy eating practices. Yet determination is not necessarily at fault. It's the brain's role as well.

It eventually becomes second nature after you've conditioned your mind to do something, including consuming unhealthily for years. Consequently, anything new that the brain appears to fight back the most is a fully revamped diet. And that is one of the explanations why it's so challenging to lose the pounds. The majority of strategies for weight loss commence by modifying the diet. Yet, in the long run, all of these dietary modifications also require much more determination to continue. So, though you could temporarily drop fat, it can come back just about as quickly.

In order to keep on track and smash all those bad eating behaviors, this segment will deliver the most successful, science-backed techniques. Here's how to break the pattern of unhealthy eating patterns.

1. Clean Your Kitchen

Whether it's your bedroom, a workspace in the office, or just your pantry, make sure you keep the spaces in your environment nice and tidy to prevent snacking excessively.

2. Prioritize Fresh Produce

It could turn into significant calorie reductions by merely reorganizing the most available foods in your pantry or sitting on your table. So, substitute this with a fruit dish after you eliminate the junk. Put fruit bowls on the table and substitute mixed nuts, peanuts, or either of these nutritious treats for those snack jars. With a bowl of Greek yogurt in the front of the refrigerator, you should also hold cleaned and ready vegetables such as broccoli, carrots, tomatoes, and bell peppers, so they are not forgotten.

3. Unfollow

Your handset is just as much a component of your surroundings in this day and era as it's also an expansion of your hand. However, when you try and start living better, that is not very wonderful news. As it plays out, it's almost as terrible for your belly to browse across your media networks to check out the sweets yourself. And if you don't need food literally, our bodies can give a message to our brains that we want to feed through the appetite hormone ghrelin. Just unfollow them if you don't want to end up consuming fatty, unhealthy foods you see in your Instagram stream.

4. Change Your Plate Size

We also consume food with our eyes as well. Food looks less as you feed yourself on a larger plate, which may contribute to overeating. Smaller dishes, on the other hand, allow food portions look considerably bigger, deceive the subconscious into assuming that you are going to eat more food than you actually are. You can enjoy more healthy meals by exchanging plates and bowls for salad plates, which can make the weight drop off your body.

5. Turn off The TV

Switch off the Screen or Netflix and turn down your music track for dinner. Or if you're out at a popular restaurant to eat, you might try ordering anything chewy! It can make you mindful of the idea that you are really consuming food, as long as you can feel the food you are consuming. You essentially fail to notice you're consuming while you're oblivious, which may contribute to a rise in food appetite.

6. Use Snack Bags

Munching directly out of a package or box mindlessly as you're still in the pantry contemplating what you should consume contributes to bingeing. This dilemma is eliminated by preparing what you are going to consume and simply sitting on a specified amount on a table. Section the things you choose to binge eat separately (and also the things you do not) to the appropriate serving amount. With a black marker, write on the package. You can also post a memo as to how many calories are in each of them.

7. Pick up A Hobby

Anything as easy as boredom can affect unhealthy eating habits and actions. You completely lose the opportunity to make good food decisions while you're tired. Rather, you now become an "emotional mess:" taking the bad dietary decisions and consuming even more than you usually do consume. According to a report of Frontiers in Psychology, you feel bored while you are unsatisfied, anxious, and unchallenged. The perfect way to defeat boredom, like planting, painting, flower arranging, needlework, blogging, listening, or climbing, is to seek stuff to do that is meaningful and stimulating. Select anything for you that is appropriate.

8. Get Plenty of Sleep

Yeah, it counts as altering the world to have those shut eyes. It's because the night shifts at the workplace might fault those who desperately want any candy and sugar-filled treats. A quick move from a table to your nice warm bed will provide you with power and result in better cognitive function such that, if appropriate, you can exercise willpower. Turn out the bulbs early in the evening to make things faster.

9. Cook At Home

From the artificial flavors to the shades of their signs, major companies have built their franchises to inspire you to buy more. These hues have been shown to draw the interest of buyers, enhance cravings, and even increase the pace at which we consume scholars at the University of Rochester claim. Drive right through the parking garage to hold your craving in line, and then eat at home. Consuming at diners typically implies little personal influence, as well as greater calorie content, regarding recipes and food preparation.

10. Do Not Keep a Stocked Pantry

The items you don't really have can't be consumed. And it is all too easy to purchase take-out or cook up a frozen meal when you are in a rush on a busy weekend, i.e., if that's all you see in your refrigerator. Experts suggest having a smaller selection of items in your kitchen, so keeping your choices restricted helps prevent bingeing, as odd as it can sound. So many options ruin the motivation, leaving you at the chance of engaging in all those chocolate bars carried in by your work colleague.

11. Become More Mindful

Giving greater care to what you eat, drink and snack on is one of the key moves in eliminating poor eating behaviors. Learn to read product labeling, get acquainted with nutrition labels, and continue to take care of all you place in your body. If you become more conscious of what you consume, you can start to comprehend how your nutrition needs to be tweaked. By maintaining a food journal, you can surely keep track of everything you eat or drink or snack on.

12. Make Plan And Be Specific

How can you begin consuming more vegetables, having timely meals each day, or go more regularly to the gym? Spell the choices down. For starters, prepare to carry a portion of fruit to the workplace for lunch each day, load up on healthy low-carb berries for easy snacks, and then go to the fitness center three times a week on the way to work. Saying, 'I'm aiming to exercise more,' won't encourage you. Talking about where and how you can work that into your schedule is what will succeed.

13. Be Realistic

Do not demand too much of it too fast from yourself. Any new behavior takes around a month to turn into a pattern. Slow and consistent, coupled with a boost of diligence, comes out on top.

14. Practice Stress Management

Work on coping with tension with training sessions, therapy, mindfulness, or something that fits for you, such that during periods of crisis, you do not slip back into all these unhealthy behaviors or use eating to make you deal with the problem.

15. Set a New Mini-Goal Each Week

Sooner or later, these micro-steps will result in big modifications. For instance, if your aim is to eat a balanced diet, remind yourself that each week you will try one different vegetable before you discover any that you'd like to eat regularly. Or search for simple ways to incorporate just one more plant option per week to your diet before you hit your target. Consider filling your afternoon sandwich with cucumber slices, incorporating fresh veggies to the morning keto-eggs you have, or loading your burger with tomatoes and broccoli for supper.

Chapter 4: What Is the Ketosis Process?

If you have searched for ways to lose weight, you might have come across this word Ketosis. Ketosis refers to a natural metabolic process whereby the body burns stored fats to get energy when there is not enough supply of glucose or carbohydrates in the body. You can achieve this by observing a low-carb diet, Ketogenic diet or intermittent fasting. These types of diets will enable your body to burn the unwanted fats in your body for energy because the supply of carbohydrates is not enough.

When the fats are broken down to produce the energy needed by the body, it releases a type of acid known as ketones that the body can excrete through urine. However, the amount of these ketones should not be too much because it will raise the acidity level in blood. This will cause a condition known as ketoacidosis that is dangerous.

4.1 How to Enter the Ketosis Process?

Reaching a ketosis state is not something that you can achieve instantly, but it can take you several hours or even days to get to that high fat-burning state. The following are tips that can stimulate your ketosis process.

1. **Reduce Your Carb Intake and Concentrate on Keto Friendly Foods**

Eating a low-carb diet will accelerate your Ketosis. Naturally, your body cells will use glucose and sugars to get energy. However, the body can also get energy from Ketones also known as the fatty acids that the liver converts into energy. Keto-friendly foods are low in carbs and high in healthy fats. You should also include high-quality protein like meat, fish, eggs, and chicken in moderation. Therefore, you should strive at eating 70% fat, 25% protein, and 5% carbs. This kind of meals will help you to stay full for longer.

You should not unless you are feeling hungry. This will ensure that the body keeps very little glucose hence you reach Ketosis faster. You will be feeling so much hunger pangs when starting, but this will reduce once you are on Ketosis. However, if you feel that hunger is too much for you, then eat Keto-friendly foods that are high in fat and have moderate protein. Remember that the portion of your meals should not increase just because you have reduced the carb intake.

You should avoid the following foods that are rich in carbs if you want to get into ketosis:

- Sweetened beverages like sodas, juice, alcoholic beverages.
- Sugary foods like ice cream.
- Starchy vegetables like potatoes, peas, beans, corn.
- Wheat products like bread, pasta, cookies, and doughnuts.
- Cereals like rice, wheat, corn, and their products.
- Unhealthy fats like margarine and corn oil

- Processed foods like canned foods or packaged fast foods.
- Avoid foods that contain preservatives, artificial coloring, and sweeteners.

Here is an example of a Keto meal plan:

Breakfast

- You can have Spinach, eggs, bacon and unsweetened coffee or tea.

Lunch

- You can have vegetable salads, meat, avocado, and broccoli and dress it with olive oil.

Dinner

- You can prepare grilled chicken, zucchini, cauliflower gratin, and some salad dressing.

2. **Increase your physical activity**

Doing physical exercises can help you get rid of stored glycogen in your body. When our bodies get busy in any physical activity, it uses muscle glycogen as a source of energy. Therefore, when the glycogen reserve decreases, the body will resort to burning fat to get the needed energy. Therefore, increasing your physical activities will accelerate your ketosis process.

3. **Try intermittent fasting**

Intermittent fasting is the trending thing for those people who are trying to lose weight. It refers to going for some hours or even days without food. When you do not supply food to your body, it will resort to stored fats to convert it into energy. This will help you in getting rid of unwanted fats in your body hence you will shed some weight in the process. There are several types of intermittent fasting. You can do the 16:8 plans, which means that you will eat within eight hours and then you fast in the remaining 16 hours. You can also go for 24 hours or more without food.

These short and long fasts will put you in a ketosis state. Although most people do intermittent fasting for weight loss, research has shown that it has other health benefits. People suffering from diabetes have found that intermittent fasting decreases blood sugar levels. It also helps in reducing cholesterol and slows down the aging symptoms. As you do the fasting, it is important to listen to your body! If you feel sick or nauseated during the fast, then you should break the fast with some healthy food.

4. **Drink enough water**

We all know that water is life! Water helps in digestion and the removal of toxins from the body system. It is also responsible for transporting important nutrients in the blood cells and other body cells. It also aids the liver in the metabolism process as well as the operations of the kidneys. Therefore, we should always keep our bodies hydrated to enable the proper functioning of the various body organs. Drinking water can also help you in your keto process by preventing the keto side effects like bad breath and dry mouth.

5. **Eat enough protein**

Although we are supposed to eat protein to achieve ketosis, we should not eat an excess of it because the body will convert the excess proteins into fats. Protein should be taken in moderation so that it can help the liver with a supply of amino acids that can be converted into glucose to be used by red blood cells and the brain cells. Proteins will also help you in building muscle mass but excessive of it will alter the production of Ketones in your body.

6. **Watch your electrolyte intake**

When you switch to a low-carb keto diet, the kidneys will get rid of some minerals and water from your system. These minerals are electrolytes and they are magnesium, salts, potassium, and calcium. These minerals are very important in our body system because without them, you will be feeling some fatigue, dizziness, cramps, and mood swings. You can find most of these minerals in the bone broth and some keto-friendly foods. You should use the lite-salt because it has both sodium and potassium in it.

7. **Increase the healthy fat intake**

Eating healthy fats will help you to stay full for longer hence it will prevent unnecessary eating. These fats or oils will help you to reach a ketosis state easily. Some of the healthy fats include:

- Avocado
- Coconut oil
- Olive oil
- Flaxseed

4.2 How to Start a Ketosis Process?

1. **Make a plan**

Plan keto-friendly meals

You can make a meal plan for a few days, to begin with. Look for keto meal plans and their recipes online. Some of the most popular keto-friendly foods are eggs, beef, vegetable salads, cucumbers, zucchini, chicken, fish, broccoli, cheese, plain yogurt, mushroom, and cauliflower among others. When preparing these foods, ensure that you use healthy oils like olive oils, coconut oils, and avocado oils.

Visit the grocery store with the keto-food list

When going shopping, ensure that you have prepared a keto-friendly shopping list. You can also search online for a keto shopping list to guide you on what to buy. Ensure that you check their labels for information about calories, fat, carb, and protein levels that they contain.

Purchase a home testing Ketone kit

It is good to measure your blood ketone level so that you can know your progress and adjust where appropriate. You can do it with the help of indicator strips or ketone meters. You should do the test at least once daily. If you are on ketosis state, the readings in your ketone testing kit should be between 0.5 mmol/l - 3 mmol/l. You can also check the ketone levels in your blood by testing the blood samples and you can request your doctor to do it.

Maintain a ketogenic diet for a week

After a few days of switching to a keto diet, you may get into a ketosis state. You can then decide on how many days you want to stay on ketosis. However, you should consult your nutritionist or doctor about how long you can safely maintain a ketogenic diet.

2. **Shift to a ketogenic diet**

Aim at consuming fewer carbs every day

You need to reduce your carb intake to less than 50 grams per day. You can achieve this by avoiding high carb foods like pasta, rice, potatoes, wheat products, corn, legumes, and beans. You can replace these foods with low-carb foods.

Eat healthy fats

We mentioned earlier that eating enough healthy fats will keep you feeling full and satisfied for a longer period. Examples of these healthy fat foods include avocados, olive oil, cheese, butter, and coconut oils. You can add these healthy fats into your keto diet to keep you satisfied for longer hours. You can also add whipping cream to your sugarless coffee or tea. Feeling more hunger pangs after switching to a keto diet is an indication that you are not eating enough healthy fats.

Avoid starchy vegetables

The vegetable is very important in our bodies because they carry very essential nutrients however, you should reduce the intake of starchy vegetables so that you can reach ketosis. You should instead eat those vegetables that are very low in carbohydrates like cruciferous vegetables (cabbage, broccoli, cauliflower, and Brussels sprouts), zucchini, cucumbers, spinach, green leaves vegetables, mushroom, and tomatoes.

Eat proteins in moderation

Proteins are very important in a ketogenic diet. However, eating proteins in excess will alter the production of ketones in your body because the body will convert it into glucose. The excess glucose will then be converted and stored as fats. A good source of protein is beef, fish, eggs among others.

Include high fiber foods in your diet

Adding high fiber foods to your diet is important because it aids in digestion. Although most high fiber foods are carbs, you can still find carb-free foods that are high in fiber like flaxseeds, chia seeds, and almonds. Eating high fiber food will help you prevent constipation.

Take more coconut oil

Using extra virgin coconut oil will help you reach your ketosis easily and it comes with other health benefits.

3. **Make lifestyle adjustments**

Avoid snacking

For optimum ketosis state, you should minimize the number of times that you eat in a day. Eating several snacks will hinder you from achieving your ketosis state. You should minimize the snack time you have per day and when you take snacks, ensure that they are keto-friendly. Avoid packaged snacks because most of them contain carbs. You can take low carb snacks like plain yogurt, macadamia nuts or a boiled egg.

Drink enough water to stay hydrated

You need to take enough water every day so that your body organs can function well. You should not drink more than enough water because it will strain the kidneys. Bone broth is also very helpful because it hydrates you as well as provides you with some minerals.

Exercise

When you engage in any physical activity, your body burns carbs into energy and if there is not enough supply of carbs, the body will resort to stored fats for energy. Therefore, exercising can hasten your ketosis process. Exercising for at least 30 minutes daily can give the best results. You can vary your type of exercise to prevent monotony. You can talk a walk, jog around or even run.

Get enough sleep

Getting enough sleep can lower your stress levels. High-stress levels can increase the level of sugar in your blood and this can hinder you from achieving ketosis faster. You should aim at sleeping a minimum of 8 hours daily. This will ensure that your body gets enough rest and re-energizes.

4.3 Why Keto Is Convenient?

Keto diet is gaining popularity because of its ability to aid in weight loss as well as enhancing the wellbeing of your physical and mental health. The following are some of the reasons why we think keto is convenient.

1. **It helps in weight loss program**

Keto diet is a low carb high-fat diet. Research shows that people who are on a keto diet lose weight faster than those other people who are on a low-fat diet. Since you will be taking high fat and low carb, you will reduce the number of times you eat per day because the high fat and protein will keep you full for longer. The reduction of carbs supply in your body will enable the body to burn stored fats for energy. This will get rid of unwanted fats in your body hence you will shed some weight because of the burned fats.

2. **Reduced blood sugar and insulin levels**

Keto has become very popular among individuals living with diabetes. This is because reducing carbs intake lowers blood sugar and insulin levels and most diabetic people confess that keto has reduced their insulin dosage by a great percentage. Research shows that the keto diet helps in controlling blood sugar and most diabetic patients who are on keto no longer use glucose-lowering medicines. Therefore, reducing carbs intake will give you good blood sugar levels and it can reverse type 2 diabetes. Keto diet has also proven to help in controlling insulin levels in patients with type 1 diabetes.

3. **Helps in treating Epilepsy in children**

A research done in 1998 on 150 children who took carbs restricted diet shows that it was effective in decreasing their seizures by 90%. The keto diet proved to be more helpful on the epilepsy patients more than the anticonvulsant drugs.

4. **Improves blood pressure**

A research done in 2007 showed that a low carb diet was effective in controlling blood pressure. This is because keto diet helps in reducing body mass, LDL cholesterol, and triglycerides. An increase in blood pressure can put you at risk of getting heart diseases and kidney failure. Triglyceride, which is the fat molecules, that circulates in the bloodstream is dangerous because it can cause heart disease.

Reducing carb intake will lower these fat molecules from your bloodstream drastically. On the other hand, LDL is bad cholesterol that circulates in the bloodstream and it can cause heart diseases. Eating a low carb diet will help you to prevent these unpleasant health conditions.

5. **Improves the mental Health**

Taking too much sugar is not good for your brain and high carbs intake has proved to worsen the condition of Alzheimer patients. Research shows that a keto diet helps to reverse Alzheimer's because the ketone bodies help in improving the memory operations of Alzheimer patients.

Ketone bodies have numerous health benefits to the brain like protecting the brain cells, preserving the neuron, and preventing its loss. Therefore, a low carb diet will significantly improve the health and functions of the brain cells.

6. **Helps in the treatment of polycystic ovary syndrome and infertility**

Polycystic ovary syndrome (PCOS) is a condition that causes infertility in most women because of the enlarged ovaries that contain cysts. High levels of insulin trigger this condition and it makes the ovaries to release androgens as well as lowering the production of sex hormone. The sex hormone glycoprotein blocks testosterone from getting into the cells. Although there is no such study that shows the relationship between PCOS and diet, keto diet help reduce insulin levels that cause PCOS. Therefore, keto can improve fertility in women.

4.4 Testing for Ketosis Process

If you are on a keto diet or fasting, chances are your body is producing ketones. However, you should be in nutritional ketosis where you will reap the most benefits. Therefore, you need to test so that you can know your level of ketosis. Keto diet alone does not determine your level of ketosis. We have other factors like your reaction to food and the activities that you engage in can determine the success of your ketosis.

Testing your ketone levels will help you to understand your progress and adjust your food where necessary. You can adjust your diet and do the testing so that you can know which kinds of food are the most effective in producing more ketones. There are three types of ketone testing:

- The blood tests
- Urine test
- Breath analyzer

The blood test will give the best and most reliable result of the three methods. Our bodies can release three types of ketone bodies namely:

- Acetoacetate: this is the first ketone body that the body produces when there is no longer a supply of glucose for energy. The liver will convert fats into fatty acids, then further converts the fatty acids into ketones. These types of ketones are present in the initial stages of ketosis and it can be detected in urine.
- Acetate (acetone): we get this ketone when acetoacetate is broken down and we exhale it through the lungs as a waste product.
- Beta-hydroxybutyrate (BHB): this is the most common ketone body that is present in blood and goes to cells in the form of energy. It provides the brain cells, muscles, and other body organs with the needed energy.

After reviewing the different types of ketones, we can now look at the various methods that we can use to test ketones in our bodies.

1. **Urine strips**

Urine strips are popular among diabetes patients because they use them to check the diabetes ketones. You can buy urine strips over the counter on any drug store or supermarket pharmacies. You will use it by dipping the strip in the urine collected and wait for a few minutes then read the color of the strip and compare it with the illustrated colors in the package. The color starts from faint to darker and the darker the strip the more ketones you have in your body.

However, urine strips do not give accurate results. This is because when entering into ketosis, acetoacetate ketones spill into the urine and this might give you a wrong impression on your level of ketosis. The level of hydration in your body will also affect the results of the strip because if you test the urine when you are highly hydrated, the results will not be the same as during dehydration. Therefore, urine strips can only give accurate results for diabetes ketones but not nutritional ketones.

2. **Breath test: Acetone indicator**

The breath test is for testing acetone, which is a byproduct of breaking down acetoacetate. However, you cannot use it to measure the number of ketones in your body that is working as fuel. You will need a breath meter that you plug into a battery source. You use the breath meter by blowing into it until the flashing light starts reading your breath acetones then you can check the color blinking and the number of times it is blinking then compare with the one illustrated in the package.

There are external factors that can alter the results of the test like chewing gums, cigarettes, toothpaste, garlic, alcohol, and other food substances that can make the sensor malfunction. Your breathing pace can also affect the acetone level. Therefore, when doing the breath test you need to consider factors like the environment condition, the breathing pace as well as the sensor validity.

You will need to practice breathing techniques severally to get reliable results. You should also purchase a breath meter that allows you to change the sensor and one that you can adjust to a known control.

3. **The blood ketone meter**

This is the most reliable method of the three. We use the blood ketone meter to measure BHB (beta-hydroxybutyrate) which is the most active ketone body, it circulates in the blood to the cells, and it converts into useful energy. You can do this by taking your blood sample through pricking your finger then squeeze the blood out onto a little strip from the machine and wait for a few seconds to read the machine. Remember to use alcohol to disinfect the area you are pricking to prevent any infection.

There you go; you can now know the BHB level in your blood! You will be able to know the number of ketone bodies that are fueling your body. The advantage of blood ketone meter is that factors like hydration or temperature do not interfere with the outcome unlike in breath tests. Although this method is expensive, it is the best way that you can know your actual ketone levels.

4.5 Eliminate the Wrong Convictions of Fat

I grew up with a mentality that fats are not healthy and that I should take a low-fat diet so that I can live a healthy life but I was wrong and I know that I am not alone in this wrong myth. The truth is that there are fats that are good for you and others are bad for your health. Therefore, the belief that a low-fat diet is healthier than a high-fat diet is not justified because it all depends on what kinds of fats you are eating.

There are different types of fats: bad ones and good ones. Monounsaturated fats and polyunsaturated are healthy fats. These fats come from vegetables, nuts, fish, and seeds. The bad fats include the industrial made Trans fats that come in solid kinds of margarine and vegetable shortening while the saturated fats are neither good nor bad and they mostly come from animal products like meat and whole milk.

Our bodies require fats because it helps in absorbing minerals and vitamins. They are also vital in building the cell membranes as well as the sheaths encircling the nerves. The belief that you should eat a low-fat diet to lower your cholesterol is also not true. The following are some of the myths about fats that nutritionist have proven to be wrong.

1. **Eating fat will make you fat**

Eating healthy fats like avocados, olive oil, coconut oil, and butter will help you stay full longer hence; it suppresses your craving for food and the urge to overeat. This can be a useful trick in weight loss management.

2. **Fats are not important in our bodies**

This is not true because healthy fats help us in absorbing important nutrients and vitamins as well as antioxidants and it supplies our bodies with energy. Fats extracted from fish, nuts, and seeds are good for the heart and the brain cells. They also help in weight loss and maintenance. Fats are also responsible for regulating body temperature and hormones.

3. **A low-fat diet is good for weight loss**

This is false. Our bodies require enough fats for energy purposes and the growth of cells. You need to know which good fats are and which ones are not good. Healthy fats like monounsaturated and polyunsaturated fats can be useful in weight loss if you include them in your diets. Most of the packaged foods that write low fat in their label contain sugars. We all know that sugar will hinder weight loss. Other factors can lead to weight gains like excess intake of carbs and calories.

4. **Fats increase cholesterol levels in the bloodstream**

Healthy fats like monounsaturated fats and polyunsaturated fats do not raise the bad cholesterol in your bloodstream but Trans- fats do and you should avoid them. You should also limit the consumption of saturated fats.

5. **Saturated fats clog the arteries**

A research done by a team of cardiologists shows that there is no evidence for this claim because they did not find any relationship between the consumption of saturated fats and the risk of heart diseases. They instead said that people should eat healthy food and exercise to prevent coronary diseases instead of blaming it on the dietary saturated fats. They also noted that patients living with chronic inflammatory disease responded well with eating healthy fats like olive oil, and the oils from nuts and fish. The omega 3 fatty acids found in these oils helps in preventing heart diseases.

Take away

It is important to know what kind of fat you are consuming because healthy fats are very crucial for healthy living while Trans fats can cause problems for your health.

4.6 Control Calories with Low Carb

Calories refer to the amount of energy that you get from food and the energy you use on physical activities. For weight gain, you subtract the calorie going out from the calorie coming in. If you want to lose weight then you should control your calorie intake even if you are on a keto diet or you can increase your physical activities so that you can burn the excess calories. The number of calories that you can consume will depend on what you want to achieve, how physically active you are and your basal metabolic rate (BMR).

Eating a low carb diet can generally reduce the number of calories that you consume because the macronutrients from high fat, protein, and low carb suppress the cravings for food. However, if you take the high-fat diet in excess, it can add up to more calorie intake. Most of the Keto-friendly foods like avocados, olive oil, and full-fat dairy contain a high amount of calories so you should eat them in moderation if you plan to lose weight.

To control the calories in a keto diet, you need to be very meticulous when it comes to your food portion. You also need to consider engaging in physical exercises to ensure that you burn more calories than the amount you take. If your plan is just to reach ketosis and improve your well-being, then your attention should be on the quality of the food you eat and not calories. However, if your main aim is to cut some weight, then you will need to watch your calorie intake and adjust appropriately.

You may not alter the amount of protein and carbs you take while on keto but you can adjust the amounts of fat so that you can monitor the caloric intake. The carb levels should be low and you can focus on the green leafy vegetables while you eat proteins in moderation to help you in building your mass muscles.

Therefore, it is important to track the number of calories that you take as well as the macronutrient's quality. This will ensure that you do not experience some nutrient deficiencies as well as gain weight from consuming too many calories. On the other hand, you should engage in physical exercises to keep you fit.

4.7 Keto and Your Health

Keto diet is among the trending diet plans available. It is popular among diabetic patients and those people who wish to lose weight. It involves taking 75% high-fat food, 20% protein, and only 5% carbs. After a few days of observing this percentage of foods in your diet, your body will get into a state called ketosis whereby the body burns stored fat in the body. Therefore, this diet plan restricts carb intake and focuses on taking a high-fat diet.

The following are some health benefits of keto:

1. **Helps in weight loss**

Perhaps this is the #1 reason why keto gained popularity. Keto helps in burning stored fats and suppressing the cravings for food so this will prevent frequent snacking. Eating fewer carbs also will help in reducing the amount of calorie intake and the protein and fat in the diet will provide a satiating effect.

When carbs intake reduces, the body's metabolism changes and accelerates the burning of fat to get energy. Therefore, the body uses most of the fat sources and converts it into energy. This process of burning fat will enable the body to burn calories too. However, to get rid of more calories you need to ensure that you limit the calorie intake and do more activities that are physical.

2. **Blood sugar control**

Keto helps in stabilizing blood sugar and the mood swings that come with the fluctuation of blood sugar levels. Keto diet is helpful to diabetes patients because the low carb intake prevents the huge spikes in blood sugar hence lowering the need for insulin. However, you should be careful not to combine a keto diet with insulin because it can lead to hypoglycemia a condition for low blood sugar. Ensure that you talk with your doctor concerning your switch of diet while on medication.

3. **Keto improves brain function and mental health**

Ketosis helps in protecting the brain from damage by shifting the energy source and regulating the energy metabolism genes. It also protects it from oxidative stress that can damage it. Oxidative stress promotes brain aging, depression, and anxiety. Ketones provide the brain with energy when it cannot get it from glucose and this helps to improve memory performance by balancing the brain chemicals.

People doing keto confess that it provides them with mental sharpness and creativity that helps them to handle multitasking while they maintain a motivated attitude. It increases blood flow to the brain hence reinforcing the various memory and sensory operations. Keto can treat epilepsy in children because of its ability to reconnect brain energy metabolism. Epileptic kids who shift to keto decrease their seizure by a greater percentage.

4. **Eliminates food cravings**

Eating a high fat, moderate protein, and low carb diet will give you a satiating effect. It will make you feel full for longer hence your appetite for frequent snacking will no longer be there. This will help you to focus on eating healthy low carb diets during the main meals. You will no longer have to worry about your addiction to overeating because keto will put your appetite under control.

5. **Reduces anxiety and depression**

Keto helps protect the brain from the damage of oxidative stress that can cause depression and anxiety. Keto diet stabilizes blood sugar that can cause fluctuation in mood swings. Therefore, being on keto can keep your moods on track!

6. **Good for your heart**

Keto can help you to lose weight that can lead to cardiovascular diseases such as high blood pressure, high blood sugar that can cause the inflammation of the arteries and increase in bad cholesterol. These conditions are not good for the heart. Therefore, keto helps in preventing the conditions that can be harmful to the heart.

Keto for Weight Loss

Keto diet is high in healthy fat with moderate protein and low carbs. Since your body will cut down the supply of carbs that is supposed to provide glucose for energy, the body will source for glucose elsewhere within the body. The liver can rescue your body with energy by converting the stored fats into ketone bodies. This process is ketosis.

To reach ketosis, you will need to restrict your daily carb intake to less than 50 grams. If you aim to lose weight, then you have to watch the calories you consume through fats. You also have to ensure that the fats that you consume are healthy ones like olive oil, avocado oils, and nuts. Remember that it is important to engage in physical exercises so that your body can burn excess calories.

Keto is a great tool for weight loss because the high fat and the protein in the diet will keep you feeling full for longer hence you will reduce the number of snack times as well as the calorie intake. Keto will help you to suppress your appetite for food giving you more self-control on what you can eat. It will also supply you with the needed energy for physical activities. Therefore, the keto diet is good enough for those people who wish to cut some weight.

4.8 The Downside of Keto

Although you can reap many benefits from a keto diet, there is an unpleasant downside of this diet plan and you should study it carefully if you plan to do it on a long-term basis. Some of the side effects occur naturally while you are on keto while others can occur if you do it the wrong way. The medical community, however, points out that keto might not be a safe long-term diet plan. Here are some of the unpleasant downsides that you will experience while on keto.

1. **Keto flu**

During the first weeks of being on keto, your body will be struggling to adapt to the new diet and the carb reduction. As a result, you will lose some water and electrolytes and this might make you feel sick. The keto flu symptoms are:

- Frequent headaches
- Fatigue

- Nausea
- Dizziness
- Brain fog
- Irritability

These symptoms can subsidize when your body enters ketosis state. You will need to press on until your body gets used to a low supply of carbohydrates.

2. **Nutritional deficiencies**

Keto diet is a restricted diet. That means there are some foods that you are not supposed to eat while on keto. The foods that you restrict or ban from your diet contain some essential nutrients to your well-being. Beans, legumes, fruits, and some vegetables provide us with vitamin C and fiber yet keto restricts its intake. Therefore, keto will deprive you of getting very important nutrients by eliminating certain food from your diet.

3. **Limited food choice**

Keto involves restriction of carbs yet most of the foods available contain carbs. If you are restricting carb intake, then it means that you will have a list of foods to choose from in your diet. You will need to cut off all the grains and their products as well as all the starchy vegetables and all the sugars. This diet plan may not be sustainable in the end because you will be craving for foods that you eliminated.

4. **Expensive**

Most of the keto meal plans are expensive compared to non-keto meals. The oils used in the keto diet like olive oils, coconut oils, and fish oils are also quite expensive when you compare to the ordinary cooking oils. You can find avocados when they are in season but the avocado oil can be hard to find not to mention its high cost.

5. **Loss of electrolytes**

When your body reaches a ketosis state, it will start eliminating glycogen from the muscles and the liver and this can lead to frequent urination. When you lose more water in your body, you also lose electrolytes like sodium, potassium, and magnesium that are very crucial for heart operations. Therefore, you will have to look for electrolyte supplements to replace the lost ones.

6. **Health concerns**

There is no existing study on the long-term safety of keto use but the medical community suggests that long-term use may not be healthy. People who have used keto for long reported digestion problems like constipation, diarrhea, and bloating. Lack of enough fiber in the diet is the main reason for such stomach problems.

Kidney stones are another common problem for someone who uses a keto diet for several months or even years. People reported to having abdominal pains that later turned to be kidney stones. This could be the effects of consuming too much animal proteins.

Ketoacidosis is also a problem that can occur while you are on a keto diet. This occurs when the body produces too much ketone bodies and the blood become too acidic. This condition is dangerous because it can damage the kidneys, liver and even the brain. Ketoacidosis can affect most people with diabetes and are on a keto diet. Therefore, diabetic individuals need to be extra watchful of their glucose levels while on keto.

Patients suffering from liver failure, pancreatitis, a disorder of fat metabolism, should consult their doctors before getting into keto. Although keto helps improve fertility in women, research shows that it can harm the growing fetus because it will lack some important nutrients that are crucial for its growth and development. You also need to check your body regularly if you have a history of anemia in your family. This is because a nutritional deficiency can put you at risk of contracting it.

7. **Weakened immune system**

Eating high fat and less fiber can mess with the balance of good and bad bacteria in your gastrointestinal tract. Since the GI protects your immune system, the imbalance of bacteria in it can have an impact on the gut-brain connection as well as the immune connection and this can cause diseases.

Fruits and vegetables are good for protecting the immune system. However, keto restricts the intake of vegetables and fruits that contains carbs this can make you susceptible to chronic illness or long-term diseases.

CPSIA information can be obtained
at www.ICGtesting.com
Printed in the USA
LVHW101519140121
676487LV00009B/613

9 781914 251030